LUCRECIA
MEMOIR
OF A MANIC
WOMAN

Introduction

o you yearn for a divine connection? Enjoy Jamie B. Goudeau, the writer of "Lucrecia - Memoir of a Manic Woman," as she learns to hear God's voice! Scripture, other people, and her own thoughts are all ways that God speaks to her. He has extraordinary ways of connecting with people, whether it is through an unexpected face in the cloud or moving music.

Aligning with this divine purpose might, however, occasionally feel like an impossible task. Jamie often finds herself entangled in the complexity of life and pleading with God for assistance. She is consistently set free by our loving and patient Father, only to become entangled once more and need His mercy to continue.

Jamie reveals her personal testimony to God's goodness and love in her memoir. It's a novel entwined with mental illness, wickedness, and promiscuity that takes the reader on a trip through misery, destruction, betrayal, sin, loss, and confusion. But its fundamental message is one of redemption, restoration, and the transforming power of God: "She, whom the Son has set free, is indeed free!" (John 8:36; Jamie's individualized quotation.)

Jamie wrote this biography to encourage you through her experience and show the incredible healing power of God. If He could cure Jamie in such a way, maybe He can heal you as well!

This book reveals Jesus Christ's amazing healing ability. Jamie has persevered through times of waning faith in a way that can only be characterized as remarkable.

Follow Jamie as she ascends from the pit of despair to the height of hope. God remained her staunch friend and never let go of her during her worst moments.

Jamie writes to help you get closer to God. She wants to show that you, too, can overcome hopelessness, betrayal, sin, loss, bewilderment, mental illness, depravity, and promiscuity by opening up about her soul and sharing God's work in her life. Jesus, who controls the utmost power of life and death, can heal you as well.

Join Jamie as she journeys through the powerful power of our Lord and Savior, Jesus Christ, from the darkness of suffering to the light of hope and healing.

LUCRECIA
MEMOIR OF A MANIC WOMAN

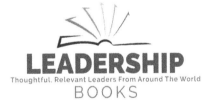

LEADERSHIP
Thoughtful, Relevant Leaders From Around The World
BOOKS

Jamie B. Goudeau

Lucrecia — Memoir of a Manic Woman
by Jamie B. Goudeau
Copyright 2023
Leadership Books, Inc
Las Vegas, Nevada – New York, NY

Leadership Books.com

For Worldwide Distribution
ISBN:
978-1-951648-44-2 (Hardcover)
978-1-951648-45-9 (Paperback)
978-1-951648-46-6 (eBook)

Dedication

I dedicate this book to all who suffer with an invisible illness like mine, whether it be bipolar disorder, anxiety, depression, obsessive compulsive disorder, post-traumatic stress disorder, or any other emotional or mental health condition.

It is my desire that by reading *Lucrecia––Memoir of a Manic Woman*, you find comfort in knowing you are not alone in your suffering, and I pray you find hope for a better tomorrow.

Acknowledgments

With a happy heart, I express my gratitude to those who helped transform this book from a mere possibility to a promising reality. As difficult as this task has been, it is not without gratefully received and highly valued encouragement. Numerous times in the past three years, I wondered if I could complete this daunting project, yet here I sit, writing the acknowledgment for *Lucrecia--Memoir of a Manic Woman*.

First, I want to give glory to God for authoring this book alongside me. It is through His inspiration and guidance that I was able to put down the words I feel will be the most meaningful to you, dear reader. I give all of the praise to You, Jesus, my Lord, and God.

Next, I want to thank my spouse, children, and family who cheered me on when I wanted to give up and walk away—especially my husband, Brent Goudeau, who has always expressed sincere belief and never doubted my abilities from the moment I first began. I love you, babe!

Last but not least, I express sincere appreciation to the staff at Leadership Books. They listened to me lament the difficulty of developing *Lucrecia*, patiently allowed me to cry tears of fear—then relief—and expressed their belief in me the entire way through the process ... all the while providing Godly support and encouragement.

I am humbled by all who gave of themselves so that the message of this book can be shared.

Table of Contents

Introduction iii

Preface 1

CHAPTER 1 "My God, what is Wrong with Me?" 5
I'm having a bad life...

CHAPTER 2 La Petite Jolie Blonde (the Pretty Little Blonde) 13
I was cute. I was little. I was a mess.

CHAPTER 3 Hidden Anger 27
Raging inferno, just below the surface...

CHAPTER 4 The Demon Within 35
The devil has gotten a hold of me.

CHAPTER 5 Lucrecia is Birthed 53
Meet my alter ego.

CHAPTER 6 God Told You What? 63
Levi, do you even know God?

CHAPTER 7 Jamie Marries the Devil Himself 75
My husband is Lucifer.

CHAPTER 8 Too Many Changes 85
Things in my life need to slow down.

CHAPTER 9 God, what are you Doing? 95
This life makes no sense to me...

CHAPTER 10 The Storm is A-Brewing 103

Warning!! Danger ahead.

CHAPTER 11 The Nightmare on the Ranch 109

It could not have been worse.

CHAPTER 12 My Second "God-Chosen" Husband 117

Jamie, you are way too gullible.

CHAPTER 13 Slow Down, Jamie 125

Can you please try to THINK???

CHAPTER 14 Another Faux Pas 133

You're getting really good at making mistakes.

CHAPTER 15 Hello Nevada! 141

Jamie is re-locating…again.

CHAPTER 16 The Investigation 147

A very scary experience for all.

CHAPTER 17 These Crazies Are God's People 157

God loves the downtrodden.

CHAPTER 18 "I am Healed — in Jesus' Name!" 171

Take care of yourself, Jamie.

CHAPTER 19 The Enemy is Among Us 185

Satan seeks whom he may destroy, we're first.

CHAPTER 20 The Beginning of the End 193

No recovery in sight.

CHAPTER 21 Another Man Done and Gone 201

I cannot keep a relationship alive.

CHAPTER 22 Score — For the Enemy 209

It just keeps getting worse.

CHAPTER 23 Sweet Home Louisiana... 221
  Returning to the sweet soil of the south.

CHAPTER 24 Is it Another Train?... 229
  I'm scared but hoping for the best.

CHAPTER 25 Jamie is Not Well.. 245
  Happier days are ahead.

CHAPTER 26 My Journey to God.. 251
  He is always there for me.

CHAPTER 27 My Journey to Healing 261
  I am learning to be there for me, too.

Epilogue 279
About the Author.. 283

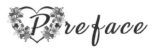

The Spider, the Web, and the Lord

Have you ever experienced the Lord speaking to you? He speaks to me! Sometimes He communicates directly—with His words —through others, the Bible, or just in my head. And sometimes, He is even more creative in the way he reaches out to me...

I may see a face in a cloud or a puddle, and God reminds me of a person to pray for or a memory of a past loved one.

I might hear a certain song and know that God is speaking it directly to my heart, or I might see something in nature that reminds me of the wonders of my God's handiwork. For example, have you ever noticed a spider's web glistening in the early morning dew? I have, and I have pondered that little spider and her web. Such ponderings have led me to these thoughts: *The little spider must be so proud of its sparkling creation after working so hard to make it just perfect.*

Such is our Father, with us, His creations. How proud He must be to show us off, "This is my Jamie, and this one is my Brent, and aaahhh, this one, he is my Jonah." Just like the spider's web, each of us is unique and different, yet we all have the same purpose: to give glory to our Father. *What a fantastic purpose!*

But is it attainable? I must say there are days I feel it is so far from my grasp—I'd just as soon give up. There are days I feel like a little spider, but rather than creatively spinning my web, I notice that I have become all tangled up and must ask my Lord for help: "Father, can you please cut this web off my legs? I seem to have wrapped myself all up and now I am a knotted mess."

Being the kind and loving Father he is, He always cuts me loose … only to find me, days later, knotted up all over again, requesting His help once more. Aaahhh, yes, I am a mess, but on — by the grace of God — go I.

It is a book about His goodness and grace. Within its pages, I have been blessed to share my story with a you— a story of defeat, destruction, betrayal, sin, loss, and confusion; a tale of mental illness, depravity, and promiscuity. But most importantly, an account of sanctification and restoration, of redemption and healing, a story of the power of God to wipe the slate clean and set me free! "She, whom the Son has set free, is free indeed!" (John 8:36; my personalized paraphrase.)

My entire purpose in writing this memoir is to allow you to experience—with me—what an awesome, amazing God I serve and exactly how much healing I have known due to His goodness, and that this will spur you to wonder... "if God can do all this for Jamie, then maybe He will do it for me too!"

I have written in order to spread the word of the real healing power that is in the name of Jesus Christ. Through the use of His spiritual forces, ordinary people, and the wonders of medical science, I have managed to overcome in a way that is nothing short of miraculous. And this healing miracle was achieved in a person who, at times, found it difficult to maintain the faith of even a tiny mustard seed.

What a journey it has been thus far! My God has taken me from the lowest depths of despair up to the mountain top again and again. He has walked me through darkness so heavy it crushed my soul. He has been with me from one extreme to another, never letting go of my hand. Always there... always.

As I pour out my heart to you, it is my prayer that you sense the presence of God while you read this record of His work in my life, and that you will seek the face of the Lord and ask Him, "What, if anything, do You have for me through reading this book?"

It is my deepest desire that I be able to point you to God through my writing. I want you to know my very soul and all that God has done in my life, to be able to share with you the deep healing I have experienced in Him and that this might touch you to see that you, too, can overcome destruction, betrayal, sin, loss, confusion, mental illness, depravity, and promiscuity. You, too, can find healing in the name of Jesus who in Himself carries the power of life and death.

May you feel His quickening grace and mercy as you descend with me now, down into the pit of pain and misery and back out into the light of hope and healing through the almighty saving power of the Lord and Savior, Jesus Christ

Chapter 1

"My God, what is wrong with me?"

A very disturbed, young wife, unable to cope, I was left at Carson City General Hospital, alone with all the crazies. I was scared and creeped-out as I looked around...

Many were crying.

One old dude with long, scraggly white hair and beard, who looked like Moses and was probably his age, was huddled in a corner chewing his fingernails. He stared straight ahead with big, wide eyes looking terrified.

A young woman, of maybe eighteen to twenty, walked frantically back and forth from the nurses' station to her room every few seconds, demanding to see the doctor for her medication. At one point she became irate and reached over the counter, swiping everything on the desk onto the floor. Papers went flying, as the file holding them came down, too, with a loud, crashing KA-BOOM! —ink pens and paperclips =scattered everywhere.

"I said, 'I want my doctor,' you retard!" she screamed at the top of her voice to the attendant.

The attendant made a Call... and then it got hairy.

"No! No! I'm sorry," she pleaded. "I didn't mean to do it. Please don't call them. I will behave, I swear, I am so sorry." She obviously had some idea of what was about to ensue because suddenly she switched from angry and out of control to contrite—even helpful—as she began to clean up the mess she has just made, getting down on her hands and knees.

But before she could finish, she was grabbed by a male nurse and put in a hold as she struggled and fought, cursing up a storm the entire time. It was like something out of a movie.

The next thing that happened really scared the living sh** out of me. As a male nurse held her in a chokehold, another nurse injected some type of medication into her arm using a huge needle—, almost instantly she went limp.

The color must have drained from my face because the attendant walked over to me and spoke very soothingly … "Miss, she's a frequent flyer," he said. "Happens regularly. She knew exactly what was going to happen and was warned each time she came to the desk. I know this is your first time here. Don't let this scare you. She just needs to sleep it off. She'll be just fine come morning. You'll see."

Sure enough, the next morning she was up and smiling and talking as though the previous night had never happened.

Wow! I won't be having any fits here. I hate needles. I just want to do my seventy-two hours and then go home to my kids. I don't belong here. These people have problems. I just need some rest and I will be fine. Lucrecia, girl, you gotta work with me here. If you show up they will never let us out of this place! Now is not the time to rear your ugly head...

... I thought to myself.

But little did I know that during my entire seventy-two hour hold period, I was being carefully observed. Apparently, the staff knew what they were doing because by the time I met the hospital's head physician, Dr. Rizzle, they had uncovered plenty of dirt on me ... and on Lucrecia, too.

When Dr. Rizzle, a short hospital white coat came into my room, his stethoscope "badge-of-office" conspicuously folded in his lab coat pocket, he smiled at me, glanced at my chart, then sat next to my bed.

"Sooo, Mrs. Jamie, tell me 'bout what bring you to Carson City General," he said in   his Hindi-accented, broken-English.

"It was all a big mistake. I am fine," I rushed in to assure him. "I just needed some rest and I feel that I am ready to go home now."

"Ahhh, so you think that it normal to have conversation with yourself at three a.m., loud so we had to put roommate in another room because you prevent her to sleep? This normal to you Mrs. Herbert? By the way, who Lucrecia?"

In shock, I looked at this doctor of Indian descent who held the keys to my freedom. I was stunned and speechless. This short, little man (who looked like an Indian version of Santa without the white beard) had silenced me.

"Look doc, I don't know what you think you heard about me, but I am fine. I was just a little confused and was trying to sort things out, and I guess I did that a little too loudly for the other patients. Please just let me go home."

Do not show your a** in here, again, Lucrecia. Stay the he** away from me right now — I want out of here!

... I again thought to myself.

"Jamie, I afraid I no can do that. Unless you tell me what bother you to you end up here on seventy-two-hour hold, I no can let you go home. You see? No?... I want believe you, but I been doing this twenty-five years. I know a thing or two about patient who end up here. You tell me when you decide you want talk and then we set the discharge date. Understand?"

We sat in silence for about five minutes. Dr. Rizzle was writing in his notebook and appeared to be unbothered by the silence. It was driving me nuts and I began to cry.

"You okay, Mrs. Herbert? Here, a tissue. I here when you ready talk."

"I just lost it! I lost my sh**," I sobbed. "I was in Louisiana visiting with my family and my husband's family and it all went downhill from there. One day I woke up and could hardly function. By the time I got to the hospital, I knew I had four kids, but I couldn't — for the life of me — remember their names. I couldn't remember the names of my children!" I thought, "My God, *what is wrong with me?*"

It was too much. I put my head down on the cold, metal table and cried loudly.

"When this begin... 'losing it?'"

I looked at him and laughed just a bit through my tears. It was all so ironic, the deep despair and frustration that bubbled up inside and mixed with my laughter.

"When did it begin? *When was it not there?* I think would be easier to answer," I replied. "The meltdown I had in Louisiana was not the first time something like that has happened to me. It has been following me all my life." I continued, "As far as I can remember, I have felt different from most people, like I had another being living inside of me who would take over and control me." I hated her. (*Lucrecia... I hate you.*) "She caused me to do mean things, say mean things, and the thoughts that go through my head would cause a demon to tremble."

"Anyone ever mention bipolar disorder to you ... or schizophrenia?" Dr. Rizzle asked.

I was suddenly inflamed. "Have you been in touch with Levi?"

"No, ma'am. I not know Levi. Obviously, you do. Who Levi to you?"

I put my head down and began to sob again. "He was right, wasn't he? He said years ago that he thought I was bipolar, and we fought and fought. I thought he was trying to smear my name. But he was right, wasn't he?"

"Jamie, who is Levi to you?"

"He is my ex-husband. I married him because I believed that God had ordained our — the — wedding and ... oh my God! I hated him. I hated him because I wanted to marry Kerri. But

Levi convinced me that God wanted me to marry him. So, I did. And I learned to hate him more. We fought and fought. And he told me that I had bipolar tendencies. I would spit on him … but he was right, wasn't he?"

I was bawling now, uncontrollably.

"What you think, Jamie? Let me read you some information about bipolar disorder and psychosis and I want you to tell me what you think of what I read to you."

Shortly thereafter, Dr. Rizzle formally diagnosed me as having a mental illness called 'Bipolar 1 disorder with psychosis.' But having a diagnosis didn't help me feel better. I was terrified of the staff and other patients there. Paranoia plagued me as I became more and more convinced the hospital was trying to kill me. I refused to eat my food because I was sure they were poisoning it.

"I can't make you eat, Mrs. Jamie," one of the mental health techs told me one day, "but you won't be allowed to leave until you do. You will have to stay here until you are better."

Yes, I'm sure you will be quite happy to keep me locked up here so you can poison me to death. Well, kill me if you must but I refuse to make it easy for any of you! "I know they are working with Tom. They are trying to poison me," I retorted. "He's mad at me because I 'decided to go crazy.'"

"Mrs. Jamie, who is Tom?" asked the tech. "And no, no one is trying to poison you. Let me show you, here I will take a bite of your food. Will you eat it then?"

"Tom is my husband and no, because they told you where the poison is, I shot back at him."

Of course, Dr. Rizzle got word of all this and came to visit me again. "You having some issue with paranoia? Anything you want tell us? Did something happen you?"

"I was investigated by Child Protective Services. It was really scary," I told him. "And my mother accused me of abusing my children. But it turned out, it was her. She let me go through that entire week of investigations and finally told me it was her. ... She had hurt my son."

I began to cry at that point.

"When you attend group, talk about this," was all he said. "It help you. Take medication. It help you."

I was given a "cocktail" of medications and they did begin to help. I soon started to feel happiness again. Something I hadn't experienced in months. I began attending group meetings sharing my childhood, disappointment with past mistakes, and my ordeal with Child Protective Services. Dr. Rizzle was right, it did help to talk, and to listen to stories similar to mine. I realized I was not alone!

I even had a divine revelation at one point. Lying in my uncomfortable hospital bed one night, after lights-out, I was feeling down and missing my kids and longing for home. I had a vision of Jesus talking to me about the people that I was with in Carson City General. He spoke intimately, lovingly... and directly to my consciousness:

"These are my people. They are the poor in spirit and are the downtrodden. They are those whom I came to save. I didn't come to save the holy and righteous ones. I came for the downtrodden, the helpless, the needy. It is no mistake that you are here with them.

You, too, are in need of help."

Suddenly these "crazy people" were *God's people,* and I was one of them.

"You got a mouthful there, Jamie-girl. You are certainly one of them, one of the crazies!" Lucrecia said inside my head.

"That ain't no lie and no exaggeration. I don't know how it is that you are twenty-eight and you're just being found out. Lord knows I have known for quite some time of the crazy! But they know now, Jamie. You can't hide it anymore — you have the certificate to prove it."

This was the beginning of a beautiful journey with my Lord. This hospital stay was an eye-opener for Jamie, Jamie the patient as well as Jamie the Mom, daughter, wife, and Child of God. No longer did I hold the mentally ill in the same light as I had before, as though they were less than or inferior humans. No! Now they were the down trodden and they were the people I was sent to help bring a healing message to...

Chapter 2

La Petite Jolie Blonde (the Pretty Little Blonde)

og gonnit, Daddy, why don't you go back to work? I would think to myself as I sprinkled the scratch corn for the chickens out in the grass on the side of the house — I was careful not to step on chicken poop in my bare feet= — you could say I was not a fan of warm chicken droppings squishing between my toes. I wished for Daddy to get back to his offshore job, where he was gone for fourteen days at a time because when he was home, he and Mom fought … a lot.

I hate feeding the chickens. I hate feeding the ducks and I hate feeding the pigs, too. That's why I just want to leave this place! All I see here are animals and grass. I hate this place!

I hated being a farm girl, to be sure. I hated the chores, I hated the animals, and I hated living in little old Faubourg, Louisiana, so far from everyone else in the world. It felt like miles and miles when in reality we were only ten minutes from the "big town" of Ville Platte. Now let me just tell you a little bit about Ville Platte so you can get a sense of just how small Faubourg is. Ville Platte is a town in south central Louisiana where the Cajun folk pass their time shooting the breeze, chewing the fat, and boozing it up on the front porch, any given day of the week. And when I say it's a small town, I mean it. When I was a kid it had no fast-food joints, not even a Wal-Mart. But Ville Platte is still bigger than Faubourg, my little nothing hometown, which still doesn't even have its own gas station, to this day.

Living in the middle of nowhere meant the only things Kay and I had to talk to were the chickens and the dogs, and so, yes, I did talk to them! I often had full-blown conversations with the farm animals. The chickens would cock their heads from side to side as if to show that I was a little off my rocker. "This one here, she has problems," I imagined them saying to each other. "*Cher*, her egg done rolled off the roof and cracked, *pauvre bete!*" (which is the south Louisiana Cajuns' French for "poor thing").

In the summers, I would get as dark as pitch from being forced to work outside all day. I had long, shiny golden blonde hair that hung down to the middle of my back, and which was straight as a stick. It was only this length because Mom and Daddy refused to allow me to cut it, which was not by my personal choice, believe that. I often wore it up in a ponytail to prevent smothering in the heat of the Louisiana summer with its *one... hundred... percent...* humidity.

Although much of my childhood was in many ways typical (if you can manage to excuse the fact that I did indeed talk daily to chickens, ducks, and even pigs),I do recall doing a whole lot of nothing with Kay (my younger sister o two years), day after long day, on that little farm out in the country on the backside of nowhere. The best times were when Daddy was gone so he couldn't fight with Mom, and when I got to spend the night at Taunte and Nonc's house, in Ville Platte.

Taunte was my mom's older sister and Nonc was Taunte's husband, my uncle … and how we loved those two. Taunte was a motherly looking woman, with ash blonde hair that she seldom fixed and kept almost as short as Nonc's. She was not much into primping, but she was very loving to me, Kay, and Nonc.

Nonc was a dark-haired man with a mustache and a full head of thick brown hair. He had a great sense of humor and loved life. Oh, how Kay and I loved them both!

Taunte was not able to have kids, so she and Nonc spoiled us plumb rotten every chance they got. Kay and I would finish up the supper dishes in a hurry when we knew they were coming over later for a short visit after supper. "Come on Kay, hurry up. Maybe if we finish in time, we can go spenna night with Taunte and Nonc." We had learned that if our chores were done, we might get to spend ("spenna") the night with Taunte and Nonc, our chance to escape the farmhouse for a weekend. Dishwater splashed and suds flew as we washed each dish with greater and greater speed and less and less accuracy, hoping and praying that Daddy would forget to check our work. We were both so young we had to kneel on the brown dining room chairs to wash the dishes. Kay sat on a gumbo pot on top of a chair to reach the sink to rinse, but we did the dishes because Daddy's train of thought was 'we weren't going to learn any younger.' It was a big deal for us to go to Taunte and Nonc's, even though they just lived over in Ville Platte, a "ten-minute drive," as I often heard Mom complain when we asked to visit. Mom was very no-nonsense and I felt, even as a kid, she was a bit on the selfish side. "It takes gas to drive there, gas money that I could spend on supper," Mom would tell us when we begged for a visit. "I have to pack your bags which means I have to do laundry. It's not as simple as 'let's go to Taunte and Nonc's house,'" she would remind us.

Mom was a short woman of medium build. Like Taunte, she wore her hair short and if she hadn't worn make-up, she could have passed for a young man some days. Daddy hated this about her and often referred to her as "Butch" because of her less-than-feminine ways. But it didn't change my mother one bit. She simply replied, "Get outta my face, you *macho pappa*." There was no love lost between them and they seldom had a nice word to say to one another. When Daddy was home from offshore, the tension between them was as thick as the gray haze in a room filled with smokers.

So we often tried to spend the night with Taunte and Nonc. It was such a welcomed change, like going to a festival.. We got to eat out either at the local Frosty's drive-thru or Nonc would barbecue chicken or pork chops. I suppose it was God's way of allowing a little sunshine with the rain in our dreary little lives.

On Saturdays, later in the evening, when we were all too tired to do anything anymore Uncle Nonc would put on the stereo under the carport, blasting Loretta Lynn and Conway Twitty as loud as possible and guzzle down one Schlitz beer after another. Once he was out of beer, he would switch to his standby, JD and Coke, in a frozen mug. "Hello, darlin,'" would fill the yard as Conway and Loretta blared over the stereo. Next came Fats Domino and Patsy Cline—and don't forget Dolly! Nonc loved him some Dolly Parton.

Looking back, I can see where my dismal childhood with parents who shared an obvious disdain for one another helped in setting up my equally dismal future with my numerous mistakes in relationships and an inability to find the right one for me…

School Is a Reprieve

As early as kindergarten, I realized that school was a place I could escape some of the troubles of home, and where I could feel appreciated. I attended Sacred Heart Catholic school where I had to wear a navy blue, white, and gold plaid uniform, which I hated, along with black and white saddle shoes. My teacher was Mrs. Regina Something-or-Other . I was a good student and enjoyed learning and quickly won the title of "Teacher's Pet," which made me a very happy child.

I recall sitting right in front of the teacher's desk and being asked to run her errands. "Jamie, can you please pass these papers out to the class for me?" It made me so proud to do this for Mrs. Regina. It was nice to have someone thank me for my help and say nice things about me. School quickly became a reprieve for me—it was at school that I learned how enjoyable it was to be appreciated! How I loved being the Teacher's Pet as I grew older, and life became harder .

I made many friends in school. I met Mary and Donna there and soon we were inseparable. I recall that we chased the boys singing out "tag, you're it." I don't know who enjoyed the game of chase more, us or the boys. I also recall spending the night at Mary's house and riding the bus home from school with her one Friday afternoon. I had such an amazing time at Mary's house, where her mom, Mrs. Renee, met us at the door with pepperoni pizza and a sponge bath toy. I remember asking her, "Mrs. Renee how did you know I was going to be here tonight?" The toy surprised me so much I think I had lost my ability to think clearly. "Jamie, a little bird told me on the way home," she said, and winked at Mary. Then we all laughed.

That weekend was great and I learned there that not all kids my age had to pluck chickens before school and that some of my friends didn't have rough outside chores to do either. This was quite an eye-opening experience for me because I thought my life was the same as Mary and Donna's something I dared not bring to the attention of my parents. Although I didn't know it at the time, my sister and I were raised much like little boy farmhands.

As much as Mom was no-nonsense, Daddy was even more so — he was even more straight to the point than her and didn't waste time with flowery words. He expected us to work wherever help was needed, both inside the house and outside with the animals. He didn't worry about our feelings, and certainly had no concern over hurting a person with his choice of words or his tone. He was, at least as far as I was concerned, a bit on the mean side. He had nothing nice to say about Mom, ever, and always had a scowl on his face. To me, he didn't enjoy his life on the farm with his family. On some days it seemed like we were his hostages more than his loved ones. And he could kill a person when he gave *the death stare* — which as a parent, he had down pat. You knew what he was saying to you just by looking at his eyes. No, he was not a nice man, but still, he was my Daddy … the only one I had.

Difficult, unpleasant parents made my home life hard. It was only at school and with friends that I felt I mattered at all. So, when I found out, at age six that my mom was pregnant again, I wasn't any too happy. My dad already played favorites with Kay, and I never seemed to get the attention I craved. A new sibling was sure to dilute their affection for me even further. *Great!* I thought, *that is just what I need. Another one to get me into trouble with Mom and Daddy.*

Feeling Like a Third Wheel

I was only two when Kay was born, so I was too young to remember her birth. All I knew was that one day I had a sister to deal with. Over time I began noticing differences in the way I was treated by my parents compared to Kay. Often, she and Daddy shared his brown recliner and she sat on him to watch TV. But if I asked to sit, the answer was, "You're too big. Go sit over yonder by your mom on the sofa." By the time mom told us she was expecting a third sibling, I was already beginning to feel like a third wheel. So, I must admit that the thought of having a new baby to compete with was not anything I looked forward to., *Why I gotta have someone else to share Mom and Dad with or have to help take care of?*

Over the next several months, I had mixed emotions regarding the new baby's arrival. I was excited... but I also felt nervous. "Jesus," I prayed, "what if my little brother or sister doesn't like me? What if they hate me? Will my Mom and Daddy hate me, too?"

I watched as the evidence of the new baby began to appear ... and my anxiety continued to mount. Mom was more and more tired as the days passed. She became grouchier, also, which was none too comforting, because she was already far from nice as moms go. I noticed my friends' mothers were always smiling and happy. Not my mom, she was ornery... and demanding... and tired.

The week our baby brother was born, Mom was trying to do the laundry but the washing machine had broken down, so she was forced to take it to Cousin Steve's trailer, which was about seventy-five yards from our front step and across the pasture.

On this particular day, she had carried one too many loads across the pasture and up four steps into his trailer. She began having pains and went into premature labor. Daddy was away at work when it happened. Our brother, Jo, was born three months early and weighted only three pounds and six ounces.

He was small enough, I have been told, that Mom could hold him in the palm of her hand. He was so tiny that even the preemie clothes hung on him so Mom put him in doll clothes. Of course. He was fragile, which freaked me out—bad. I just couldn't imagine anything being that small, other than the tiny beagle puppies that Nonc and Taunte's dogs had earlier that summer.

I worried daily as Jo had to stay in the hospital in New Orleans for months until he was strong enough to come home. This broke my Mom's heart, and my heart, and Kay's, too. I'm sure that my Daddy's heart was also hurting, but I can't say for sure because he didn't say much about his feelings from one day to the next... unless he was mad, then he cussed – in French. You knew he was mad if he began speaking in French, and it was not nice what he was saying, I learned later.

Jo finally grew strong enough to be released from the hospital. It had been a long time coming and we were all so relieved on that special day. Indeed, he appeared just as Mom had described him for us as he lay in the hospital.

"He is so small, Boog (her pet-name for me). His small baby arms are like little crayons and his tiny toes are miniature raisins. He is no bigger than one of your dolls. Even his cry is gentle and soft. He sounds like a little puppy whimpering when he cries."

Jo had gray-blue eyes and light-colored hair. He was perfect and he was precious, and we loved him instantly. It was a great day when he came home; I felt Jesus had answered my prayers of bringing my baby brother home safely to us.

I loved my little brother and he became more of a blessing to me as each day passed. I learned to be a little mommy, changing his diaper, feeding him, and often rocking him to sleep. It was like having a real live baby doll to take care of. My heart melted more and more each time he looked at me with those shiny gray-blue eyes. On the day he smiled at me for the first time, I was so excited it was better than getting a new toy. Kay and I often fought over Jo (we fought mostly over being able to get that feeling from mothering him).

Jo brought such joy to our little farm. Suddenly there was something new happening from one day to the next. It was no longer simply the dark and dreary same ol', same ol'... at our house. It was exciting to see what he was going to learn. He was smart and noticed everything, so we did too.

But as great as it was to have Jo in our home, it changed nothing between my parents. They continued to fight and argue and threaten one another. Their relationship was a dark cloud that hovered over all of us and never went away.

Daddy's way of saying hello to mom when he got home was something like, "Why can't you clean this dam*** house so that it doesn't smell like a pig's stye when I walk in? You can't get off your lazy good for nothing' a** long enough to pass a rag on the furniture and a mop on the floor?" To which Mom would reply in the same "loving" manner: "You Macho Pappa, why don't you bite me? I had sh** to do today and you can pass the mop your own dam*** self if it bothers you so much." Then next we would hear the screen door slam, BAM, and the tires' screech as Daddy peeled out of the driveway, scattering rocks everywhere. Upon his exit, Mom would often plead with him, "Please don't leave. I need you here. We need you here."

But it never stopped him. He was gone before the last word was out of her mouth. I knew that she was hurt because she would cry after he left. She tried to hide it by crying in her bedroom, but I could hear her.

That made me sad, and I was angry with Daddy. He was wrong for treating Mom that way. *Afterall,* I reasoned to myself, *she stays home and takes care of the house and Jo all day. She can't do everything!* Their fights gave me little reason to feel warm fuzzies for either one of them, but especially Daddy.

Jesus, Save Me!

She was short and round and beautiful with fair skin and sparkling blue eyes. She had long, light brown hair, which was frosted with a hint of blonde that she wore up in a very well-done bun. She listened to my mother and let her cry...often.

As usual, I was in the kitchen listening to the adults talk, while Kay and Jo were playing out in the living room with Todd and Carl, Mrs. Joy and Mr. Jude's boys. Without warning, tears began to roll down my cheeks and I sobbed uncontrollably. This was an ugly cry, you know, that cry when your face is all red, your nose is running like a drippy faucet, and your shoulders are shaking? Yeah, that cry, that's the one – right there in front of a house full of people... in the kitchen, my mother, and Mrs. Joy – and in the living room – Mr. Jude, Todd, Kay, Jo, and Carl. They all looked up at my outburst.

Surprised by my reaction, Mom wiped her tears and came around the table, wanting to know why I was crying. I couldn't answer her – I didn't know why I was bawling. I just sat there with tears running down my freckled cheeks and a lump in my throat – I couldn't speak.

Mrs. Joy walked over to me then and held me close. She wiped my tears and began to witness about the Lord Jesus and His power to save and to heal.

"You know beautiful, Jesus can heal your broken heart," she said soothingly. "He can take away all the pain you are feeling, and He can put joy in your hurting heart. He makes me feel better when I am hurting. Would you like to know Jesus as your Savior, Jamie? I think He is speaking to you."

"Can I be saved right now?" I asked, wanting to have Jesus in my heart.

"Yes, Jamie, you can! Just close your eyes and repeat after me, 'I am a sinner and I ask You, Father God, to forgive me for my sins and wash me clean. I invite You, Jesus, to become Lord of my life and to come and live in my heart. Change me and make me more like You. Amen.'"

I gave my heart to Jesus right then and there... in Mrs. Joy's kitchen, my little skinny arms raised in the air and tears flooding my face. Oh, how I needed a Savior. Yes! I needed a Savior. Now I had Jesus who was my Savior and God, who spoke to me every night.

I needed Him in my life in a real way. He was going to save me.

That experience was the beginning of a much stronger relationship with my Lord. I had always known of God, but now He lived inside of me, and I knew that I had access to Him at all times. Considering what I had lived through, that meant a lot to this once-lost country girl from Faubourg.

Fix That Bob-bin (Pouty Lip, in Cajun French)

Even after asking Jesus to come and live in my heart and save me, I still felt parts of my soul were missing, and my heart was broken.

But like anyone who comes from an unhappy home, I learned from a young age how to fake a smile in public. "Jamie is always smiling. She is such a happy child" people would comment to my mom. They had no way of knowing that my smile was my mask. I hid the pain behind my supposedly happy demeanor.

At home I was often chided for being sad, so I learned that no matter what kind of pain I was feeling on the inside, I needed to smile... and I tried to, at least most of the time.

On the occasions I wasn't able to grit my teeth and pretend very well, my mom would often say things like "Go to your room with that lip. I don't need to see that *bob-bin'* [a pouty lip, in Cajun French]. Go and don't trip over your big lip on the way to your room. Don't come out until you have found your smile and fixed that sour face."

It did nothing to help me to like her. I remember thinking to myself: *Why you gotta be so mean? You can't even ask me why I am sad.*

The only time I had anything nice to think about my mother was when I was thanking God for my little brother and that it was because of her that Jo was in our lives. *You are really a great mom, high five on that one, really, way to go!* I would think to myself, almost sarcastically.

When I needed refuge from the storms of life, I put my time and energy into Jo. He was an angel sent from heaven to brighten our small, dismal world. His sweet smile and gray-blue eyes helped warm pieces of my cold heart and brought life back to the deadened parts of my soul.

So, this is how life was on our little farm while I was a young girl. I guess it easily could have been worse and I am truly grateful for the Lord's mercy in preventing that...until it did worsen...And then I thanked Him for his presence in my life.

Chapter 3

Hidden Anger

Angry? Was I angry? Naw, not me! I was a happy child…or was that smile just a façade? Was my smile a way of hiding the pent-up emotions that needed to be hidden from the rest of the world? Perhaps so…but in my defense, I had reason to be angry and—I had reason to keep it hidden as well…

Although I loved Jo and he was such a blessing in my life, as I grew older, I learned to resent Mom for the amount of time she expected me to spend with him. Daddy was often away, either working or drinking at the local bar so Mom was left to see about us and the farm, which meant that there were plenty of chores to do, inside and out, and taking care of Jo was one of them.

I would whine to Mom in the most pathetic voice I could muster… "Ewww, why do I have to change his diaper again? Can't Kay do it this time?"

"Your sister is still too small to change a poopy diaper. You do as you are told, or I will get the belt to your little bottom. And stop your whining."

Angry and disgusted, I would stomp off to find the diaper bag, rolling my fiery green eyes into the back of my head as soon as I was safely out of Mom's sight. I was approaching eleven by this time, and Jo was going on four. He was yet to be potty trained, and though Mom had explained in the past that because Jo was a preemie, he would be delayed in meeting some milestones, I wasn't always as accepting of his slow progress—I guess you could say, changing his poopy diapers was not my favorite chore! Sometimes I had to dig deep to find patience.

As I approached my teenage years, I noticed that my anger towards frustrating situations in our unhappy home just continued to accelerate. I had a hard time hiding it. My parents just chocked it all up to puberty and changing hormones. I, too, thought that maybe it was just the fact that I was maturing. But later I would learn that hormones were not the cause of the extreme feelings of rage and frustration festering inside me— it was much more serious.

All I knew at the time was that I was an unhappy child and since my parents were also unhappy, I blamed them and took things out on Kay. We got along on some days, and then there were the days we tried to tear one another's hair out by the handful. Yes, I do mean that quite literally and I recall throwing things across our bedroom at her and Jo. "Get out of my room!" I would scream at both of them. "I don't want you in here. I am trying to be alone, stupid!"

One day Jo ran to Daddy and told on me. He yelled at me from his brown recliner, where he always sat to watch the evening news when he was home. When I heard the tone of his voice, I knew that I had made a *faux pas* that was going to cost me. I was waiting for the switch, but that didn't happen. When I got to his recliner, he was waiting for me with his green-eyed death stare. He glared as he spoke: "Jamie, what the hell were you thinking? You get on your knees right here and you will get up when **my** knees hurt. How do you like that?" My Dad always did have a way with words...

I was so humiliated that I hated him all the more at that moment. "I didn't mean to hit him. I just wanted him to leave my room," I told Daddy, fighting back tears.

As I knelt there, I began having terrifying thoughts: *I am not like the others. I am not like Kay or Jo. I am different from my friends. My anger is worse. It's like the devil lives inside of me. I scare myself from the rage I feel. I could really hurt someone at times, and I don't think I would even care.*

This was one of the first times this demon-like thing that lived inside me seemed to rear her ugly head. That "being," whatever it was, felt so real to me that I wrote a poem about her:

Inside of me, it lives
I cannot control it.
Inside of me, it breathes.
I cannot control it.
I feel it, but I cannot see it.
It lives in me, but it is not me.
Who are you???

I overheard Mom talking to Taunte one day on the front porch of our home about my anger issues. They were both in agreement that it had to be hormones because they had no other rational explanation. But I wondered to myself at that young age, what

29

exactly were hormones and how were they to blame for my anger?

As I matured, I of course had hormones, and they did cause problems for me, but anger wasn't one of them. The problems caused by my hormones were with my emerging desire for the opposite sex.

It started early for me, at age ten, when I met my first love at Mrs. Joy's house. His name was Kerri, and to me, he was the most good-looking boy I had ever laid eyes on. The fact that he was a city boy from the outskirts of New Orleans only added to his appeal.

Kerri was Mrs. Joy's twin sister's son. He had light brown wavy hair and sea-green eyes with long eye lashes. I loved his olive skin and New Orleans accent that matched his Aunt Joy's. He and Mrs. Joy's son, Todd, were very close and he introduced us.

We bonded quickly, Kerri and I, and we often talked about God together. He, too, had accepted Jesus Christ as his Lord and Savior and had been saved as well. This was comforting to me because none of my friends knew God as I did. But Kerri had a relationship with Him like mine.

We seldom spent time with one another because of the great physical distance between us and he only came to visit in summer months and possibly holidays. The distance didn't make any difference to my heart. I loved him.

When we could spend time together, we talked for hours about our love for music (we both liked some rock, country, and some Christian rock, too), our disappointments surrounding our family life, and our desire to live closer to one other so we could see each other more often. I loved listening to Kerri's accent. He reminded me so much of Mrs. Joy with his Creole twang and the way he stretched his words.

I kept my love for Kerri a secret. I didn't share it with anyone. But, as the years passed, it became harder to hide.

When he came to visit Todd at Mrs. Joy's house during the summer, we were inseparable. Mom and his Aunt Joy took us all to do things regularly and we loved our time together, splashing and swimming at the city pool or at Lake View Park, walking the trails at Chicot State Park, and riding my Welsh pony named Pocco. It helped the summers to pass by a little faster when Kerri came to visit. I always looked for a hint of him at Todd's house: the mention of him coming to visit, the family's car … anything. I just wanted to be where he was as much as I could.

Then when he finally arrived, Todd would call and say, "Guess who I have sitting in my room?" Although I never said a word to anyone about him, everyone who knew us could see that Kerri and I were crazy for one another, even as young kids.

I counted on Kerri during those wonderful summers to help me cope with the troubles at home and when he would head back to New Orleans my dismal life would start all over again. How I missed him!

He had promised to write, and I couldn't wait to hear from him. Every day I ran to the mailbox to check for a letter from Kerri. Finally, it arrived!

I read the words of his letter until it was worn out, the edges becoming frayed and torn. Eventually the words were too faded to read. But that was okay because by that time I had it completely memorized.

Dear Jamie,

I miss you and since we can't talk over the phone, I am writing to you. I have been thinking that you could be my girlfriend if I didn't live so far away. I hope that you think of me sometimes. I listen to the song, "I've Been Waiting for a Girl Like You" and I think of you.

I hope to see you soon!

Kerri

I so loved how different Kerri was from all the boys in Faubourg. He was never one to waste words and got right to the point. He had great stories to tell about city life and all the fun things to do there. He often shared how he went to the video arcade and played games for hours on end. That sounded great to a small town country girl!

But even with all that city excitement, I started to get the feeling that Kerri was lonely. He would tell me, "Jamie, you spend time with your mom and daddy every day. You and your family eat meals together. It's not like that at my house. My parents are busy all the time and I am given thirty dollars and told to go to the arcade so my parents can get work done."

What he didn't understand was that it was lonely at my home too. I was lonely even in the middle of the supper table with my entire family surrounding me. I often felt like an outsider in my family. The anger that raged inside caused me to feel as though there was a huge barrier between me and my siblings. And as for my parents, neither one ever noticed how isolated I felt from everyone. They were too busy yelling at one another to worry about me.

I Just Want Outta Here!

Although I listened to Kerri's complaints about his life in the city, I still longed to go to New Orleans (a hundred and sixty miles southeast of Faubourg), or anywhere else *other* than my small, boring hometown.

Kerri and Todd, on the other hand, loved coming to our farm to ride Pocco around our never-ending property, which seemed to stretch from one end of Faubourg to the other. "Man, I love riding your horse," Kerri would tell me. "It's a blast. I love it here Jamie! I feel so free when I make Pocco run, and the wind is whipping through my hair. You are so lucky!"

But the Brown family farm was old and mundane for me. I just wanted to be in the city. I wanted to see the lights and hear the bells and whistles. I wanted adventure! Kerri would shake his head as I complained about wanting to escape my dull life.

"Kerri, have you ever been so bored you found yourself talking to farm animals?" I asked him one day. Well, I have! I've had full-blown conversations with chickens and ducks. So, don't talk to me about how boring your life is in New Orleans. You have no idea what boring is, dude. And don't ask whether the farm animals replied to me. That is a conversation for a whole 'nother day."

I knew, from a young age, that I had way too much creative energy to have it stifled by the nothingness of my dismal country life in Faubourg. The clock seemed to tick backwards there—I think some days in that town there were forty-eight hours! It often drove me insane, and I resented my parents for my awful existence. "I want excitement and adventure. I want to see the world. I want to LIVE!" I cried to Kerri. He just didn't understand what he had. He had the life I wanted. He had excitement. It was hard loving someone who lived so far away, but my heart knew no distance...

Many boys took Kerri's place when he was in New Orleans. But none of them ever came close to him in comparison. It was only their proximity that drew me to them—we could talk and hang out since I couldn't even call Kerri because it was long distance and "that cost money."

But very few of my relationships worked out as a teenager. Each time Kerri would come into town, I would find a reason to dump my boyfriend-of-the-moment and get over to Todd's house...

Kerri's short visits were, in my opinion, God's way of allowing me a little sunshine into my dark and dreary days. When he was around my heart smiled and my anger subsided. But, when he was gone, I was left to cope again. As his visits became fewer and farther in between, my ability to cope waned. Sooner or later the anger would be an issue for me. That much I knew.

Chapter 4

The Demon Within

You never know what lurks beneath the surface. You never know if a smile is genuine. This I learned about myself as time passed and I grew older and saw Kerri less and less. I smiled on the outside, but there was an evil force brewing on the inside of me that I was having a hard time taming until I met Will. He would help me tame the demon within (or so I thought).

My love for Kerri never went away, but the fact that he lived miles away really made it hard to think about anything serious with him.

As I got older, I had way too much self-confidence (or what I thought was confidence at the time) and too little understanding and use for tact to stay emotionally hung up on someone who lived miles away.

In my freshman year in high school, age fifteen, I met Will. He was a junior and heavily involved in athletics, he was good at both baseball and football. Will was just getting over a breakup with one of my classmates, and I found him to be handsome and funny, and I decided that I liked him within minutes of meeting him. He had dark brown eyes and straight, jet-black hair, and I was drawn to his easy-going style and great sense of humor.

Because he was a little on the reserved side, he struck me as safe, and I liked that. But I thought he could use some help coming out of his shell. I gave him time to come around to the idea of asking me on a date, and finally, after weeks of hinting, I gave up waiting and *asked him*.

He laughed and said, "Well, I don't have to wonder if you're shy."

"Nope, not when I see something I like," I answered without hesitation.

I guess Will liked that answer because he took me up on the offer, and we soon became an item.

On the bus ride home one day, after learning about Will, Todd asked me, "Jamie, what about Kerri?"

"What about him, Todd? You know he lives in New Orleans, and the only time I hear anything from him is when he is here, and that ain't often at all. I need someone who is here, and besides, I like Will a lot."

Todd loved to stir the pot between me and Kerri.

"Well, it's just as well. You know Kerri has many girls from New Orleans he hangs out with," Todd replied. "I never wanted to tell you, but he almost has a new girlfriend every week when we talk."

"Well, I hope he is happy... because I know I am."

Though I said this to Todd, inside, my heart was broken. I suspected Kerri had many other girls, but I didn't need to hear about them from Todd.

I think while dating Will, I almost managed to put Kerri out of my mind. But I must be honest, he was never far from my heart. I still loved him. Will or no Will, I loved Kerri. We lived too far apart to be an item, but my heart refused to let go of him.

Jamie, you know you are so wrong for the way you feel about that city dude. You need to leave it alone. When was the last time you heard one word from him? He has your phone number. He could call you, but he doesn't. Ever! I would think to myself. *Besides that, you have Will, and he's a good guy. He is good to you and is there for you when you need someone to cry to, and he loves hanging out with you. Let it go, you idiot! LET IT GO!*

Though Will and I dated all through my high school years, I never did let go of Kerri, but I learned to love the one I was with. I was lucky enough to attend all four proms—with Will. But, spending so much time together, it was impossible to hide "my inner being" from him. We fought, and I would scream and throw things at him, and…threaten him.

My angry outbursts would go something like this: "Why were you dancing with her? You want her? What are you doing with me if you want to dance with her?"

"Jamie, I don't know what you want from me or how to please you," he would complain. "No, I don't want anyone else but you. But I also have other friends and you sure dance with other guys. Get over yourself, would you?"

Will would try to defend himself and calm me down, but most of the time, I wasn't having it and would pout for hours. I blamed my jealousy on every girl that he danced with, talked to, or made the mistake of glancing at. The poor dude was in a no-win situation because if he danced with other girls, I was angry, but if he was near me too much, that made me feel as though he was smothering me.

"What a hypocrite you are, Jamie! Here you are in love with another guy and still giving Will ten kinds of he** for simply being friendly. Come on, girl! Wake up!" I scolded myself. I knew better, but the evil force inside of me refused to let me alone.

But that was classic Jamie behavior. I excused myself, even justifying and rationalizing how I treated him.

Jamie, you're not wrong for loving both Kerri and Will," my mind would tell me. *"You can't help what your heart feels. It's how you treat Will that matters. You're faithful to him, and you never try to contact Kerri. You have even tried to forget him. Don't beat yourself up over it.*

But I couldn't let it go, and that, too, angered me. My fierce feelings were becoming out of control the older I got and the more freedom I had away from my parents. It was beginning to scare even me.

It was then that I began to suspect that this anger stemmed from the many disappointments in my life, including the loss of Kerri, my parent's behavior, the way they made me feel unimportant and unwanted, my home life, all of which had never been dealt with. And poor Will regularly got the brunt of my fury and rage. It wasn't fair to him, this I knew, but I was not able to control it either—like the time I screamed uncontrollably at him after a date, during which I felt he had spent too much time watching the Louisianna State University (LSU) football game and not enough time with me- "What is the matter with you, Will?" I shrieked. "You are more concerned with your football games than spending time with your own girlfriend! I don't even know why I bother with you. You make me sick!"

I'd pushed him—hard... but he pushed me back—harder: "Jamie if you ever push me like that again, I will lay into you like a dude. Understand me?"

I cried, but he had made himself clear. I was putting myself in a man's shoes, and I deserved his response. I did have enough sense to know when it was time to chill because I had crossed the line. This was one of those times. So, when Will dropped me off without even so much as a goodbye hug, I sucked it up.

Of course, my volatile temper didn't help our relationship, and we broke up a couple of times. One time was the summer of my seventeenth year—that summer was great because I spent it with Kerri. We were together every moment I was not working, and he was not with Todd. We went to Chicot State Park, walked the Arboretum trails, and enjoyed swimming at Lake View Park. But, as usual, Kerri left to go back to New Orleans, and I was left to my dreary life in Faubourg.

Even through the separations, Will and I always managed to find one another. We were inseparable at times, and then there were times that we couldn't stand the sight of one another, where Will spent most of his time trying to put up with me and my awful temperament.

Will never complained to anyone about me despite how terrible I was to him. I hated myself for the way I treated him, but I made excuses for myself because, after all, "all couples fight." You would think I could have realized my relationship with Will was going to end up like my parent's if things didn't change, but for some reason, I never worried whether Will would be there for me. Even when we broke up, I felt certain that, at any given point, I could get him back. Yes, that's the misplaced over-confidence I mentioned earlier—it wasn't a pretty thing.

Under the Stars

Four years into our stormy relationship, on a mid-August night, Will took me to the Steamboat (a fancy romantic seafood restaurant) just outside of Ville Platte in the quaint, antique town of Washington. We sat out on the back deck on that beautiful star-filled night, chatting and laughing, having a great time, as we often did when we weren't at each other's throats. Then Will became very serious and asked if I trusted him, and I laughed and said, "Of course I trust you. I wouldn't be here if I didn't, I assure you that!"

"Then close your eyes tightly until I say to open them." I had no idea what to expect, but I closed my eyes, as he requested. Then I heard him say, "Okay, now you can open them."

When I opened my eyes, he was down on one knee, in front of me, holding a small black box in the palm of his hand, which held a stunning marquis diamond ring.

"Jamie, you have given me some of the best memories of my life and I am so blessed to have met you. I would be honored if you would allow me to be your husband and if you would be willing to be my wife. I love you, Jamie. Will you marry me?"

I looked down at Will on one knee and heard myself answer, "Yes, Will, I will marry you." But my heart was elsewhere, and my mind was having other thoughts: *Yes, I will marry you. But you will never be Kerri! You are simply a replacement, a fake, a decoy, to distract me from the pain of not being with him.* Inside, I must admit, I desperately wished it was Kerri down on his knees proposing to me but just as quickly as the thought entered my mind, I dismissed it. Kerri was nothing but a distant fantasy. Will was a very present reality.

Yet Will's presence wasn't enough to resolve the inner turmoil I felt as I fought to put Kerri behind me. He had been a bright spot in my life—a source of happiness and a refuge from the darkness. But he was also an elusive fantasy. My immature teenage heart hadn't realized yet that the relationship would never amount to anything lasting or significant. After all, he never contacted me when he was in New Orleans—I was simply a pastime when he was visiting the Faubourg area. I needed to realize that, and I needed to accept it.

I prayed silently and intently to the Lord for help: "*God help me. I cannot do this on my own. Please heal my heart and help me to let him go. Help me to be the wife to Will he deserves, and thank you for putting him in my life.*"

After that prayer, I made a sincere effort to focus on Will and leave Kerri behind once and for all.

Over the next eight months, I focused all my energy and extra time on planning our wedding. I realize now that I should have been happy, but I slowly became increasingly agitated. Will called it "pre-wedding jitters" and tolerated me as best he could, having patience to the extreme … "Yes, Jamie, we can have a rainbow wedding, even though you know that is not what I would rather. Yes, the guys will wear matching cummerbunds, does that make you happy?"

And it did make me happy until I heard songs that Kerri and I had listened to together, and then I would be terribly distracted. I got really good at ignoring the red flags. I had resigned to myself that I was going to marry Will, although I was in love with another guy. It never occurred to me that I should break it off with Will or that I was being unfair to him. Well, yes, I guess it did occur to me, but never enough that I felt like I needed to act on it. I would simply push the thought out of my head and focus on the task at hand (the wedding).

Will and I planned a huge Catholic affair at Sacred Heart Catholic Church in Ville Platte. I was paying for the biggest part of it while Will focused on preparing a rental house for us to live in. I was so glad that I had a full-time job at Wal-Mart and that they allowed me to take overtime because this huge wedding was going to cost a small fortune.

My parents had divorced while I was in high school, and Mom had moved to Texas and wasn't working, so she was unable to help. Daddy had agreed to pay for the alcohol (which was a big help), but it was pretty much up to me and Will to pull everything off.

'Geez, Louise, why does everything have to cost so much?' I cried to myself repeatedly as I slowly made all the arrangements

over the next eight months. And even though I was checking the flowers, food, band, and photographer off my list, I still couldn't get a handle on my nerves. But it was coming along nicely, and I was beginning to picture it on May 20, 1989.

Flowers.	Check.
Band.	Check.
Food.	Check.
Dance hall rented.	Check.
Church booked.	Check.
Dress bought, (it fit)	Check.
Cleaned	Check.
Pressed	Check.
Photographer contracted.	Check.
Honeymoon booked.	Check.
Rehearsal supper planned.	Check.
Nerves intact.	... **No!**

Will and I fought about the details and cost of the wedding, but he often gave in to me just to prevent another fight. I suppose he got tired of all the demands, though, because, at some point in our engagement, he began to fight back. And fight we did, into the middle of the night at times. We would fight at our rental house, at my grandmother's house, where I had moved after graduation and my parent's divorce. We would fight whenever and wherever I had a notion to become angry. Finally, he had been pushed to his limits and sometimes would become so angry he got threatening: "No! I won't drive you home! You can walk! ... And I hope you get raped on the way!"

The Demon Manifestation

Our relationship was fast becoming a toxic one and I must admit I was largely to blame. I couldn't help myself. It was the thing that lived in me.

It was the psychotic Jamie, who refused to lay low and refused to behave. I hated her. She annoyed me and was going to cause me to lose Will if she didn't chill the he** out! This demonic thing inside of me had been tormenting me for years and now was tormenting Will, too. I tried my best to cope and manage it, reasoning with myself, doing deep breathing exercises, taking long hot bubble baths, and exercising daily. But still, it refused to be tamed.

I had friends tell me, "Jamie you're going to lose Will if you don't lighten up. He won't stick around forever if you continue to treat him so badly. He is so good to you. He sends you roses for every anniversary; he buys you anything you ask for if he can afford it, he is there for you when you're upset. What more could you ask for?"

I knew it was true. I couldn't deny what they were telling me. So, again I would try so hard to kill the devil that lived in me. But somewhere in my heart, I think I knew what the problem was. It wasn't simply anger. It was deeper than that. It was a broken heart that refused to heal. …

Why, God? Why?

On a hot, sunny Saturday afternoon, e a few weeks before the wedding, I was at Wal-Mart checking out my groceries after a shift, tired and so ready to chill for a few hours before a date with Will later that night.

My feet were pounding (I always wore strappy flat sandals and then paid for it later) and I had a headache to boot. I looked up as I grabbed my keys, and it was then that I noticed him … there staring at me from across the service desk counter was no one other than Kerri himself. I had not seen him since the year prior. *Like a ghost from my past!* I found myself thinking.

Our eyes met and a **thousand megawatts** *of power* pass between us, like a lightning bolt on steroids.

First, time stood still. I felt the blood drain from my head. My legs suddenly felt like they weighed five hundred pounds. I stood there motionless, unable to breathe. My heart began to race what felt like at a *hundred and fifty miles per hour.*

Seeing him again was way, *way* too much. I had to escape! I had to get the heck out of there. I ran out of the store, leaving all the groceries I had just purchased on the check-out counter. *Wal-Mart can have them – I need air!* I thought wildly.

Once in the parking lot I could hear a male voice, in Creole twang, calling to me loudly from behind, "Jamie, wait. I just want to talk to you. Wait!"

Kerri had grabbed my groceries and was running after me. My hands were shaking, and I was saying to myself, "*This is not supposed to be **happening**, Jamie. You are not supposed to be **this shaken** by him. **You're engaged to Will**.*"

I tried to get into my car to leave before Kerri could get to me, but I couldn't get my keys into the door lock fast enough. My hands were shaking too badly, and I couldn't see through my tears. Kerri ran up to me and handed me the groceries.

"You might want these," he said. It was more than I could take, and I began to cry and shudder. I stammered and crawfished backwards, flat up against my car.

Kerri stood in front of me, his long, tanned, muscular arms around either side of me, his hands on my car, trapping me against him and the driver's side door.

He was still every bit as good-looking, with his olive skin, sea-green eyes, and wavy light brown hair. It was too much … seeing him. He was killing me and had no idea how deeply he was shooting arrows into my heart.

He could see that I was shaking and quickly took a step back from me, reaching out to steady my groceries, and giving me some breathing room. "Jamie, I didn't mean to upset you. Why are you crying?" he asked, gently lifting my chin with his fingertip, forcing my eyes to look into his. They were sincere and full of concern, but he appeared to be oblivious to his effect on me.

"I was shocked to see you," he went on, "and then when you ran out of the store, I realized that you were upset. I was with Aunt Joy, and she pointed out the groceries you left behind and said to me, 'Go after her,' so I grabbed your bags and ran after you. You're still as beautiful as I remember."

He didn't look in the least bit flustered.

"You just don't understand what you are doing t' … you can't possibly understand what you are doing to me," I almost whispered in reply.

To which, he looked totally confused.

We hadn't seen one another or spoken in over a year, since the summer of my junior year. He had no way of knowing that my heart still belonged to him.

He took my hand and put it on his chest — instantly I got a little light-headed. Desperately I juggled the grocery bags.

"My heart is beating so fast. Do you feel that?" he asked me. "I have missed you. How are you? Are you happy? I hear you're engaged?"

He was sucking the breath out of me with each word.

"Yes, Kerri, I am engaged to Will," I managed to say, taking my hand back. I stared down at my shoes and didn't offer to show him my ring. "I have to be somewhere … I need to go. I will be late. … Thank you … ugh, I mean thank you for carrying my bags to me."

"Jamie, we haven't seen one another in over a year. Can't you stay and talk a few more minutes?" Kerri pleaded with me. But it was more than I could deal with for even a moment longer. I had to go.

"No, I can't … I'm sorry. I need to go. … I have to get the cold stuff into the … ah … fridge."

I drove off, leaving him standing there, obviously confused by my behavior. I wept bitterly the whole way home, tears flowing from my eyes like somehow a giant faucet had suddenly been turned on in my heart. I was crying so hard, I had to pull over at one point, onto the side of a backroad. I felt like my heart was going to explode, it hurt so deeply. I cried out to my God in pure anguish. There were so many conflicting emotions that I thought I had dealt with. Boy, was I wrong!

"Whyyyyy?" I screamed at Him, pounding my fists in fury on the steering wheel until I exhausted myself and collapsed into a fiery mess of twisted emotion—sobbing without restraint—allowing the last few years of pent-up pain to flow through my body.

"How could you allow this to happen to me, Jesus?" I half screamed; half prayed. "Don't you remember, I prayed and asked you to help me to let him go? How could you do this to me? How … could … you? Don't you know how hard this has been for me? I loved him. I STILL LOVE HIM!" I was so emotional in that moment I didn't know who I was angriest at … myself, Kerri, or God.

"What was that back there, anyway," I continued, "like you decided to dangle him in my face to remind me of what I am missing? Was that Your way of toying with me? Was it some kind of sick, twisted joke, huh God?'

Then I felt the Lord answering me through the voice of His Spirit, who lives within me: *"All Kerri wanted to do, Jamie, was to be polite and bring the groceries you left on the counter as you ran out of the store. Are you pleased with yourself? Are you pleased with how you handled that situation? You did it to yourself. You know you want him. You know you still love him with all the capacity you can actually love another human being. So, don't blame God! God didn't run out of Wal-Mart. You did that, Jamie!"*

With that, I shut my eyes, laid my head on the steering wheel, and sobbed helplessly and shamelessly. I cried until the tears refused to flow anymore. I cried until my mascara had smeared all over my face. I cried until I was emotionally depleted.

It must have been at least thirty minutes later when I started the car and slowly made my way home to my grandmother's house, completely exhausted and emotionally numb. I fixed my make-up and ran into my room to avoid questions about my swollen, bloodshot eyes. I was not in the mood to talk to anyone.

Seeing Kerri like that ended up being a turning point for me— he had no idea of how much he had changed my day... my future... my life.

From there, things only got worse for me emotionally. I couldn't shut my heart up for a second. No matter how hard I prayed for the strength to let Kerri go, my heart flat refused. I ached for him, yet I hated him. I hated the control he had over me, even from miles away, without even knowing that he was hurting me, with no idea just how much I was still in love with him.

Jamie is Jilted

Will must have sensed something had changed in me because less than two weeks before the wedding, and about two months after that encounter with Kerri, he asked if we could rethink things. He took me to a restaurant to break it to me gently, and as we sat holding hands, he quietly said, "I have been thinking about us, and I feel that we need to hold off on the wedding. I just think that we need to be sure before we get married. We fight all the time, and that is not the life I want; not with you; not with anyone. This has been on my mind for weeks. And today, I sat in church and prayed. I felt I needed to tell you I cannot marry you, at least not right now. Please try to understand."

"What do you mean you can't marry me?" I asked incredulously. "I have been planning this wedding for months. What am I supposed to do with everything? Sell it?"

"Jamie, I know, and I will pay you back, but I just cannot do this right now. I know it was God's voice telling me to break it off. I'm sorry."

"God's voice? You heard *God's voice* telling you to break it off? God *spoke to you*?"

"Yes, Jamie, He did. I am sure of it. You are not the only one He talks to, you know. We have been fighting for months, and I just can't live that life. My parents have fought all my life, and I can't live that way. And your parents did the same thing to you. Please try to understand. I just need some time. I am not saying it's over, but I need some time."

We broke up that night after a heartfelt conversation that went well into the morning hours. I didn't expect it but for the first time in months, I felt a sense of relief. Finally, I was free from having to live a lie. I never told Will about Kerri, but I went to bed that night and apologized to God.

"Lord, you know me and know my heart. I am so sorry for being so angry with you. I see now that You were trying to prevent me from making a huge mistake. I was going to marry Will while being in love with Kerri. I was so wrong. Thank you, Father, for saving me from a horrible mistake."

But instead of feeling God's soothing reassurance that He accepted my prayer, I heard the demon thing speak to me, chiding me, berating me, tearing me down. *"There ... are you happy now, farm girl? You can't even hold onto a dull boy from the town of Ville Platte. How do you think you would have ever captured and kept the attention of a city guy like Kerry, who lives an exciting life? You are something else ...."*

I cried myself to sleep that night.

The next day Will came with me to tell my family members. They took it harder than I did, I think. As you would expect, there were many tears and condolences shared, but I knew in my heart it was the right thing both for me and Will.

The only thing left to do was grieve the loss of our plans to live our lives together. I cried most of my tears alone with my God, at work, while driving my car, at night in bed, wherever they hit me. I knew I had to grieve to get past it. And grieve I did.

The demon had won out once again. It was a never-ending battle for me where happiness was concerned and I had myself to thank for that, myself and the evil that dwelled within me. It refused to allow me to feel peace and it was worsening as I grew older. What was this thing? Was I possessed? No! Jesus lived in my heart. Then was I evil? No! I knew I was a good person. But what was it? What caused me to be so vile and hurtful to those I loved? And what could I do about it? That was the million-dollar-question at this time in my life as I grieved my relationship to Will, fought to forget Kerri once and for all, and found happiness to be elusive…

Chapter 5

Lucrecia is Birthed

If you had known Jamie back then, you wouldn't have been surprised to know that it didn't simply end. Did you really think that with all that anger welling up inside of me that I would just go away quietly and allow Will to dump me without recoil? Ha! Not about to happen! Jamie and Will were about to have one last hoorah!

About a month after the breakup, I was driving past Will's house on a Sunday afternoon after attending church on my way to work, singing along to a song on the radio, smiling and enjoying the beautiful sunny day—totally minding my own business and feeling pretty good, despite the pain of being jilted two weeks before my wedding day.

As I drove by his house, of course, I glanced over at it. In his driveway, I saw the car of a mutual female friend parked there. Instantly I became enraged, my blood began to boil, and I had tunnel vision. I slammed on my brakes and threw the car into reverse, never thinking that I could have dropped the transmission right there on the roadway or bothering to check for any traffic behind or around me. I screeched into his driveway, dust clouds swirling and rocks flying as my car stopped just short of his front steps. I stomped up the steps and pounded on the screen door. No one answered. I could hear voices (both male and female), so I knew that he was home, and that Nikki was there as well.

After knocking at least three times and getting no response, I had an impulsive fit, throwing open the screen door and trying to open the front door. Of course, it was locked. So, I did what any girl in my situation would have done, right? I balled up my fist and stuck it right through the glass in the door, reached in — blood dripping down my arm — and unlocked the deadbolt, letting myself in. Glass lay shattered all over Will's living room floor as I entered the house.

The first thing I saw was Nikki sitting on the sofa, stunned and pale from shock. Will sat across the room in the rocker recliner, glaring at me.

Nikki and I locked eyes for a moment, and then finally, she screamed in utter fear, "Oh my God! Will, I need to leave. I need to go now."

She had probably seen the devil staring at her, right out of my eyes and into hers and down into her soul — that same devil that had been tormenting me for years, the one who was about to be unleashed on her. At this point, I'm quite certain I was frothing and foaming at the mouth. It was not a pretty sight.

Suddenly, I heard the demon, a disembodied voice inside my head, *"No, Nikki dear, you don't need to leave. You need to stay right there and let me rip your head off your shoulders. You have no idea of what I am capable of … but I am fixing to show you! Why don't you stay so we can play?"*

Now totally embarrassed from the scene I had created when I saw the obvious innocence on Nikki's and Will's faces, I ran into the bathroom and began to clean my arm, which was still dripping blood from being ripped open by the broken glass, reluctantly I came out of the bathroom and faced Will and Nikki. "Nikki, don't go! I'm sorry! I promise you I will not hurt you!" I begged her, red-faced and humiliated. I couldn't believe what I had done. I was appalled by my actions. "I will go. You don't have to leave."

In my head, I heard, *"No, Nikki, I'm not going to hurt you. Not at all. It won't hurt when I rip your head clean off your shoulders. Naw, you will only feel it for a few seconds. Come on, buttercup! Stay!"*

After Nikki made her very quick exit, I turned to Will, who was furious with me. "What is the matter with you? Have you completely lost your mind!!?"

This was a side of Will I did not know. He was fed up and embarrassed at the scene I had created.

"Look at what you have done. My door is broken, the glass is shattered, and I guess I am going to have to repair the damages, as usual, and clean up your mess!"

I stammered as I backed up, now scared of the look on Will's face.

"I... I knew it was her car," I said in a shaky voice. "I knew you had feelings for her. The whole time we were together, you had feelings for her, didn't you? What the hell was she doing here when we just broke up a few weeks ago? No! I haven't lost my mind. I just want to know what the heck she is doing here."

"That's the problem, Jamie Marie. You! You make me crazy! You had me so confused that she was here talking to me about our breakup to help me to clear my head—as friends do." Pointing emphatically at the broken door, he yelled, "So, get out of my house, NOW, and DO NOT come back here! You are either crazy or demon possessed, I don't know which one, and I don't care either. I don't want anything more to do with you. I've had it! Do you hear me, Go NOW!"

I didn't know what else to do. Only hours before, I had been in church, asking the Lord to give me strength to overcome the grief. Yet here I stood, covered in blood, and standing in a pile of glass—I had really messed up. I could see in Will's face that I had crossed the line and knew him well enough to know that there would be no going back.

I left Will's house, and if our relationship hadn't ended before then, I had surely nailed the coffin shut that day! *What were you thinking? You were in love with Kerri and going to marry Will anyway, then you lose your mind because he is talking to a friend?* I berated myself. *What is wrong with you?! What an idiot you are at times! That girl means nothing to Will! How in the world can you be so jealous when you're in love with Kerri anyway?'*

I was completely out of control. The demon who lived inside me—Lucrecia—was fully born that day. There was no going back; she was on full display. I couldn't pretend any longer that she didn't exist; I couldn't shove all her madness under the rug anymore; I couldn't hide her anywhere; I couldn't kill her—she had made a complete and undeniable appearance, and there was nothing I could do, at this point, to fix any of it.

Am I mad? I wondered. *Am I not seeing the enormity of my mistakes?* I wasn't sure I really wanted to know.

I was so disappointed in myself for what happened that day. Not only did I fully lose Will's friendship, forever, but I lost Nikki's as well, along with a few other people. Of course, they took Will and Nikki's side, feeling I needed help, refusing to befriend me until I sought it out. The problem was, even though I agreed I needed help, I wasn't ready to seek it out just yet.

And that's where the big trouble started. I began detaching myself from "Jamie," speaking of myself in the third person, attempting to put a deliberate sense of distance between me and Lucrecia (or the "Jamie" who had bewitched me).

Jamie, Stop Yo'self!

But weeks later, I was lying in my double-sized comfy bed at my grandmother's house on a Saturday night and heard Foreigner on the radio singing, *"I've been waiting for a girl like you...."* Without warning, my heart and mind were filled with memories of Kerri. I had fought the urge to think of him previously because I had been with Will. But now Will was really gone... I let the Kerri-thoughts flow. I wondered how he was doing and how he had been spending his time. I could hear the twang in his voice clearly in my head. Then, I began to wonder if he was still up.

Earlier in the year, Kerri had joined the military and was serving at the army base in Fort Hood, Texas. Without thinking, I called information and requested the number to his base. Next thing I knew I was on the phone with the base operator:

"Kerri? Yes, he is on his way back from New Orleans. Sure, I can give him the message that you called, Jamie. No problem."

Two minutes to midnight my phone rang. It was Kerri!

I was breathless.

"Jamie, I was driving home from seeing Jeanie (Kerri's girlfriend who he had been with since high school), and my family and I heard Foreigner singing; I've *been waiting for a girl like you*," I heard him saying. "All I could think about was you and then I get to the base, and they tell me, 'some girl from Louisiana called. I think her name was Jamie.'... and I was like, 'Jamie from Louisiana? Did you get her number?'"

Thank you, God, for answering the cries of my heart, I found myself saying to Him. What were the chances of Kerri and I listening to the same radio station on the same night and hearing the Foreigner song at the same time, thinking the same thoughts? It had to be the workings of my God.

We talked into the early morning hours, reminiscing, catching up, and sharing memories. Time seemed to stand still for me. My heart exploded with a mosaic of emotions as I lost myself in the intoxicating sound of his Creole accent. Nothing had changed between us. Time had passed, but everything was the same as it had always been—sweet and enduring.

Two hours into our conversation, Kerri sounded very sleepy, "Jamie, I need to get some rest, sweetheart, but it was great talking to you. Where are you staying now? Are you still out in the country by Todd? Give me your new address, and maybe I will come over sometime, okay?"

After we hung up, I lay there with my heart pounding out of my chest. It took me quite some time to drift off to sleep. I was way too keyed up with the love I felt for him. Though it had laid dormant in obedience to my will for some time, it never died, and with that realization, I finally drifted off to sleep.

Is It Really You?!"OH MY GOD! KERRI, IS IT REALLY YOU?" I screamed without shame as I watched a black Ford truck drive into my grandmother's driveway later the next morning. I was out of my mind excited! No Christmas present ever could have compared to having Kerri show up in Faubourg that July morning in 1989.

He stepped out of his truck in his army fatigues and military haircut and instantly took my breath away. Tears filled my eyes — I was engulfed with so many emotions. I went from happiness to excitement to joy to pure love and back to happiness. Yes! I still loved Kerri, who had stolen my heart at age ten and was still laying claim to it nine years later.

I ran to him the same way I had always done whenever he had come to town for a surprise visit. We sat in his truck bed and listened to the radio and talked and talked and talked.

He told me about his new girlfriend and how disappointed he was in the relationship because they fought all the time, and that she was so demanding. I told him about my failed relationship with Will and how he had ended it because we constantly fought as well. "Jamie, I have missed you and our talks. We can talk about anything or nothing at all, and we still enjoy one another's company. I have never found that with another girl, ever. It is so special to me. You are special to me."

Tears filled my eyes as I said this to him, and he quietly wiped them away. It was a magical moment...

After hours of waiting to hear it without asking, I finally said to him in a scared voice, barely above a whisper, "Kerri, I have to ask you, do you love me?"

He stopped talking and became very still and serious. He drew in a deep breath. He propped himself up onto his elbow so he could look down into my eyes. He looked at me with pure tenderness and sincerity, then said very seriously, "Jamie, I have *always* loved you, and *I always will* love you. No matter what happens... today or in the future... *I will always love you.* Believe that."

I had yearned desperately to hear those words for years! When I thought of him, there was no other that could compare! My heart had steadfastly refused to let go of him, and now here he was, telling me that he loved me. I think that I died at that moment, and the angels carried me to heaven, and I just wanted to stay there.

I leaned in and gently kissed him on the cheek and replied, "I feel the same way, and you have no idea how long I have waited to hear those words from you." If I could have frozen this moment in time and put it in a box for safekeeping, I would have done it.

Kerri stayed most of the day and then told me that he had to get back to the base. "Jamie, I need to go. I have training for the next three weeks, but I will be back. I need to speak to my girlfriend and tell her about you, about us. Please wait for me. I promise you I will be back, and we will discuss where we go from here. Thank you so much for calling the base. I don't think I would have been brave enough to reach out to you because I felt that you had decided it was over between us. I am so glad I was wrong."

Just before he drove away, he said to me, "You do know that I am engaged? I will have to break things off with her. This changes everything. I don't expect that there will be a wedding now."

"Kerri," I gently replied, "there can still be a wedding. I will marry you."

He stopped then, dead in his tracks, turned around, and walked back to me as I stood in the driveway, "Jamie, are you proposing to me?"

I giggled nervously at the intensity of the moment and said, "Well, yes, I suppose I am. I love you. I have loved you ever since we first met. I would happily marry you."

He paused for a moment, staring intently at me, "I will break it off with her. Just wait for me. You will not hear from me in a month because I will be in training, but I will be back. I love you, Jamie."

I watched as Kerri drove away that sultry Monday evening in July until his black 4x4 was no longer within sight. Back in my bedroom, I rehearsed over and over the day's events—the moment he said he loved me, playing it over and over in my head.

I counted down the days until he would return from his month of training.

But all the while Lucrecia was persistently whispering in my ear. "*So how are you going to ruin this, Jamie? This is your chance; your dream is finally coming true. But it is well known you can't hold onto anyone. Eventually the crazy wins! Give it up sister. You should know by now that you can't hide me. You know you've tried. You tried with Will, and it never worked. Eventually, you showed him what a psycho we truly are. Don't deny it! Don't even try to deny it.*"

And she would not stop, she continued, "*You know the crazy is there. It's there when you pray, it's there when you smile, it's there when you are nice, it's there when you are relaxing, it's there no matter what. It may be subdued. It may even be kind enough to lay dormant for a while but know this sister: It never dies...we are psycho... we are psycho... we are psycho... psycho.... psycho....psycho!*"

Chapter 6

God Told You What?

*I*t was a glorious time, being in touch with Kerri again, so why did I feel with all my heart that Lucrecia was going to ruin it all? Surely, I was just being paranoid, right? Surely this time was going to be different. I had to believe this!

The following Sunday, even though it was only day one of Kerri's twenty-eight-day training, and I knew it would seem like forever before we could be together again, I went to the small Assemblies of God church in Ville Platte, where I had been attending without fail for the last five years. It was a Protestant church—spirit-centered and spirit-filled.

This particular Sunday, I walked in and barely noticed a uniformed Marine standing near the doorway. I was not impressed with his appearance or military rank and felt no need to introduce myself to this newcomer, so I walked right past him and to my seat with Mrs. Joy. After the service, while I was gathering my things to leave, I felt a tap on my shoulder; I turned to see this Marine from the back of the church.

"Hi, I'm Levi." He said as he reached his hand out to shake mine. I shook his hand and said politely, "Hi, I'm Jamie; nice to meet you. Did you enjoy the service today?"

Yawn! I really was not interested in talking to him. He appeared to be stuffy, and it was obvious to me that he was full of himself. He stood straight as a stick, and his uniform looked like it had just come out of the cleaners. He was not my type at all.

"Yes, I enjoyed the message," he answered. Can we talk for a minute?" I was ready to leave, so I said, "I'm really in a hurry. Can we chat another time?"

Persistently he told me it wouldn't take long. "Can I just walk you to your car?" I agreed, then hugged Mrs. Joy and kissed her on the cheek, "tell Mr. Jude, Todd, and Carl hi for me. See you next week. Love you."

As we walked, Levi proceeded to tell me how he had heard that there was a young woman in the congregation whose fiancé had broken it off with her, and, he wanted to meet her. He wasted no time in getting to the point: "I believe that God spared you for me. I believe that you are the wife I have been waiting for, and that is why God had your fiancé break it off with you."

Amused, I stopped right where I was, threw my head back, and laughed at him. *Who is this dude?* I thought in disgust. *Like, is there something seriously wrong with this guy? God talks to me! I don't need an errand boy to do His bidding.* I turned to him and replied rather briskly, "Oh yeah? Well, I'll tell you what—when God tells me that, then we can talk. Are you done? Because I need to go now. I have to get to work."

With that, I drove off. I didn't even look back or give the conversation with Levi another thought; how I wish that I had kept that attitude. It would have saved me a lot of heartache later on.

The following Wednesday (day nine of Kerri's twenty-eight-day training), Levi was there in church again in his Marine Corps uniform. He smiled at me as I walked through the door and went to my seat on the third row for an evening worship service.

This time Levi took a different approach. He introduced himself to my mom after the service, who had just moved back to Ville Platte from Texas. They stood after the service and talked and talked. He learned from her that she was looking for a job. As I was walking up to get her to leave, I heard him say, "I'm looking for someone to manage my restaurant in Bunkie. I'll train you. Would you be interested?"

From that moment on, my mother and Levi became thick as thieves. They spent hours together, both at work and after work. The funny thing is, after she spent time with him, I began noticing that she was constantly giving me the third degree, asking me things like, "What kind of things do you like in a guy? When is Kerri going to come back for you? Are you planning to marry him?"

Blah. Blah. Blah.

Feeling fed up and frustrated, I told her, "If Levi has questions about me, why don't you tell *him* to ask me *himself*? Or is he too scared?" I stared right into her eyes, daring her to deny it.

She blushed and turned away, a little taken aback by my directness. "Well, he likes you ..." she replied. "Why don't you go out with him? He's a nice guy ... I think you'd like him. At least think about it ...."

I was silent, so she went on.

"Look, I know how you feel about Kerri, but, Boog, you haven't seen him or heard from him since he came for a few hours on that day, a week ago. Don't you think he could find five minutes to make a phone call to you? At least Levi is here and is showing interest."

This made me angry because she had never liked Kerri. She gave no explanation as to why, but in my opinion, she'd never given him a chance. Now that I think about it, she never liked Will, either. In fact, Levi is the only guy that she ever seemed to approve of out of all the guys I had introduced her to.

And that should have told me something. *Duh! Here's your sign!* I should have turned and run as far and as fast as I could from her and him. But I had never been one to think past the nose on my face when it came to guys. I lived my life from one moment to the next and was pretty carefree and spontaneous. In short, I was young and stupid!

Maybe it would be okay to let someone spend a little money on me. What could it hurt? Besides, it has been a couple of weeks since I've had any male company. That just won't do.

"Tell him to call me. I'll think about it," I said finally.

What was wrong with this picture? I had only just recently been dumped by my boyfriend of four years, had Kerri on hold for two weeks with a possible proposal, and was now telling my mother to have this obnoxious, pushy military man give me a call? I'm not sure why it never occurred to me (or to her) that there was something seriously wrong with all this.

"... Next?"

The very same day, I was sitting in the living room talking to my grandmother about my boring day when Levi called me on the house phone.

"Hi, Jamie, it's Levi; I was just wondering if you would consider letting me take you for a ride on a plane. I am a trained pilot."

I hadn't expected that and impulsively decided that a ride in an airplane wouldn't be so bad. I had been bored for days, and I was never one to deal well with boredom. What could it hurt?

Surprisingly, Levi was very polite and well-mannered. He opened the car door for me, as well as the restaurant door, where we went out to eat before the ride. I was not used to that from anyone I had ever met! We had a fun time, and I was very shocked by how much I actually enjoyed my time with him. For a minute, I forgot all about Kerri.

After that, it was pretty much a flurry of dating and spending time together. Every day we would see each other. We listened to Petra. I learned to jog. We ate at the restaurant he managed in Bunkie. I drove his car, a stick shift. There was never a dull moment, and I liked that about him.

After church on the following Sunday, one week into Kerri's twenty-eight days of training, Levi laid a real doozy on me, telling me at my grandmother's kitchen table that he had been given a prophecy that promised him a chosen wife. "Jamie, she has been saved for me. I truly believe that the Lord spared you from marrying your ex-fiancé because you are to be my wife."

Again, with this story? I didn't know what to think at that point. I had been enjoying my time with him, and so all this had taken me by complete surprise.

I replied to him, "If I am to be your wife, Levi, you will know things about me that I have only shared with God. He will tell you these things, and you will be able to confirm my reservations by revealing these things through the Holy Spirit."

Without missing a beat, Levi began surprising me with things he suddenly "just knew" about me, such as the fact that the mauve and mint green placemats in his kitchen were my favorite (a fact I had never told him). He invited me to attend a Christian concert with him, which I had wanted to go to but had never talked about with him. By the end of that week (Kerri had been gone three weeks by then), Levi had me convinced that he was hearing from the Holy Spirit.

Jamie is Engaged, Again

August 4th, 1989 (twenty-six days into Kerri's twenty-eight-day training), again sitting at my grandmother's kitchen table, Levi poured his heart out to me tearfully. He shared that his brother had found and married his wife within six weeks. "This is a dream come true for me. I want to marry you, Jamie. I want you to be my wife."

By this time, I was convinced that, indeed, the Holy Spirit had been talking to Levi. How could he have known those things but by God? (It couldn't have been my mom, right?) It had to be God's will—just as he had said.

So, I said, "Yes, Levi, I will marry you."

Without blinking, he gave me a small diamond ring and a promise, "I promise you that by the time we are married, you will have a proper ring with a proper diamond set in it."

Squealing, I ran into the living room to show Grandmother and Mom the ring. "What's this?" they both asked, somewhat surprised. I replied, "We are engaged. Levi has asked me to marry him, and I have accepted."

I'm not certain of who was more shocked, them or me. This was the Marine that I had no interest in even introducing myself to just weeks prior, and now I was agreeing to marry him.

It had been a whirlwind romance, and Levi pushed for a quick wedding. "I want to get married on September 16. Does that give you enough time to plan our wedding?"

"Oh my gosh, Levi. That is six weeks from today. Have you lost your mind? I can't plan an entire wedding in six weeks."

It was August 4, only twelve weeks since Will had broken off our wedding and only two days until Kerri came home from training—you think perhaps I may have been confused?

"Jamie, let's do a small wedding. Just our family and a few important guests. It can be done. I know it can be done. I believe in you."

Mais, it will have to be small because my pocketbook surely cannot afford much, I thought to myself. *I surely hope you plan to contribute, Mr. Marine man.*

So, off to the drawing board, I went, taking my mother with me. I had a wedding to plan and a short amount of time to plan it.

A few days later, Levi and I were sitting in his car in Grandmother's driveway after going for a jog. We had the skylight open and were both kicked back, enjoying the stars. But as relaxed as I was, I had been worried all day about something, so finally I just spit it out... "How are we going to pay for this wedding?"

I had paid for my last wedding, which ended in disaster and was not about to ask my parents to help pay for another one.

Without hesitation, he replied, "You told me in one of our previous conversations that you have money saved from not using all of your student loans. I think this is God's way of providing for our wedding. We will use that money, and I will help you pay it all back."

Levi had it all figured out.

He had all the answers.

And that is what kept me snagged within the whole Levi scheme—God must have been in it all because everything seemed to be falling into place.

Except for one giant detail … Kerri.

It hit me suddenly (though I don't know why or how I had just up and forgotten it before) that I had made a promise to Kerri just four short weeks earlier to take him as my husband.

Kerri … only five days after accepting Levi's proposal, was knocking on Grandmother's screened front door. "Is Jamie home? I need to speak with her, please," He'd returned.

Parking his black 4x4 behind Levi's car, he was back and asking to speak with me. My heart was in my toes as I prepared to walk out of the house to face him.

"Do you need me to come with you?" Levi asked. I'm sure he was fearful that I would change my mind once I was face-to-face with Kerri again, the love of my life.

"No. I need to do this alone," Thank God I had at least that much common sense about me. I went out to face him. "Jamie, I came as soon as I heard. Todd told me. I had to hear it from you! Tell me it isn't true. This is a small town, and people lie, and gossip starts. Tell me you are not marrying another man. Please tell me you are not, and this is all some misunderstanding."

But before I could answer, Kerri bent down to grab my hand and saw the engagement ring Levi had given me.

"What in the heck is this, Jamie?" he demanded. I did exactly what I said I was going to do. I broke it off with my fiancé as soon as I got back from visiting you. She has been begging me to reconsider, but I knew that I loved you all along and told her that. "Then Todd told me, 'So have you heard? She's engaged to some Marine guy who she hardly knows.' I thought he was joking with me. Then Aunt Joy confirmed it.

'Yes, it's true,' she said, 'she just met him in church, and they're engaged to be married on September the 16th.'"

Kerri was crying by now, which was tearing my heart to shreds.

"Jamie, it was like a thousand arrows through my heart when I heard the news, and I had to see you." Then I saw this green Stanza in the driveway, and I knew that I had been made a fool. "*Why* Jamie? Have you lost your mind?"

I looked at him and in my deluded state, I said, "Don't worry Kerri. I have never loved anyone as I love you and I will never love another man the way I love you. But I have to do the Lord's will, and sometimes that means sacrificing what you want for what He wants."

"Jamie, you are making a huge mistake," he pleaded with me. "HUGE. You don't even love him. You can't possibly love him; you just professed your love for me and now you're going to marry *him*? I believe you have truly lost your mind, just like Aunt Joy was telling me. This is it between us; it is over. Do you hear me? When this doesn't work out—and I assure you it won't—DO NOT CALL ME. I am done with you. You will *never* have the opportunity to hurt me this way again. I do *not* understand what is wrong with you."

And with that, he walked to his black 4x4 without even so much as a backward glance and drove away.

I never saw nor heard from Kerri again after that day. But I was convinced that it was God's will for me to give him up, the love of my life, to marry Levi. No! I didn't love Levi. I was head over heels in love with Kerri. But more than I loved Kerri, I loved

God. And if I had to sacrifice my will and my heart to do God's will, I was going to do that. I would not live in rebellion against God.

Chapter 7

Jamie Marries the Devil Himself

It is amazing how quickly a wedding can come together when the enemy is helping to plan it.

I found the perfect dress at a store in Lafayette on sale at a price I could afford. "Yes, I love it," I said, with little birdies flying around my head.

I remember smiling the whole way home and Aunt T telling me, "You will make a beautiful bride in your chosen gown."

Mom had agreed to pay for the flowers for the wedding, and Daddy was paying for the rehearsal supper, though he was none too happy about my choice of a groom. He had made that perfectly clear to both Levi and me. But again, I was not concerned about his feelings. I was more concerned about serving God and doing His will.

I quickly booked the honeymoon based on something Levi had said, "The beach is one of my favorite places, Jamie." Okay, Cancun it is. Four nights and five days, "where the sun will be shining and the water will be clear and beautiful. I can't wait to see it, Levi. I'm so happy you enjoy the sun and beach; I love it!"

The wedding plans flew together, and in a matter of five weeks, everything had been finalized and pretty much paid for by me, except the few things my parents had agreed to provide, The guest list had to be shortened quite a few times to accommodate what I could afford. It was going to be a small quaint wedding with family and a few close friends. ...

The day finally arrived—September 16, 1989—and indeed, it was a beautiful day. A slight crisp breeze and a hint of autumn, which was just around the corner, stirred the air. The sun was shining without a cloud in the sky, which I had fervently hoped for since it was a garden wedding at the Arboretum in Bayou Chicot.

I remember asking Daddy shortly before the ceremony began if he was nervous. He was going to walk me down the aisle, being the dutiful father. "I am just ready to get this sh** over." He said abruptly.

I was used to his disdain by now. I could hardly expect anything else from him. "Well, thanks for being so happy for me," I replied just as shortly. That was the end of that conversation. It normally would have upset me, but I just let it roll off my back. This was my day, and he was not going to ruin it for me.

The music began, and he walked me to Levi, who was dressed all in white and sweating from head to toe. It was a romantic ceremony and went off without a hitch. Everything was beautiful and perfect. Levi and I had written our own vows and had memorized them and said them to one another with all sincerity. We kissed, marched out, and had a very nice reception.

Then, it was off to Cancun, where everything went straight to hell...

The Honeymoon from Hell

I could vomit at the thought of that horrible trip to Cancun. It was truly awful, and that is being kind. Levi became sick from the heat of the sun, which was something he had known was going to happen. "I hate the sun. I always get sun sickness."

He had lied to me. *Why had he said he loved the beach if he couldn't even be in the sun?*

I was furious about this and the money I had spent on a ruined honeymoon. *This man is so unbelievable. First, I have to pay for the wedding. Then if that's not enough, I also pay for a honeymoon that I can't enjoy because he lied to me. This is just great, Levi! Just unbelievably fantastic! I just cannot believe this sh**. This ought to be a great life if it's starting out like this.*

"Levi, we talked about this, and you said you loved the sun and the beach. Why didn't you tell me? I spent a small fortune and now you can't even enjoy it with me."

"Just go to the pool," he said, "and I will meet you there later."

But "later" never came. He stayed in bed with a fever and chills for the first two days. I spent time running back and forth between the pool and hotel room afraid that he was going to die but torn by my desire to enjoy my hard-earned trip.

On the third day, he woke up fresh and alert and announced to me as I was getting dressed for the day:

"I am feeling better today. I think that we should go sightseeing in Mexico. I feel that Mexico is something you need to see."

I had no idea of what horror that outing would bring to my world. It was a total culture shock for me. I had never in my life seen such poverty and deplorable living conditions, people living in grass huts with dirt floors, with no running water. There were babies in the streets begging for water or money or food, with flies buzzing around their dirty faces. Their mothers were nowhere to be seen.

The roads were dirt and filled with potholes, and every pothole; it seemed, had at least three to four Mexican babies in it, trying to escape the heat of the sun or drinking the contaminated water from it. I was shocked beyond imagination to experience this, and on my honeymoon, nonetheless.

I knew Levi had arranged the whole Mexican "honeymoon" on purpose, to be cruel to me. He was unkind beyond words, and in Cancun —I was only beginning to see what he was capable of.

"You needed to see this, Jamie. You have never left Louisiana to see how other people live. You need to understand the horrors of the world. You are much too naïve."

"How could you do this to me on our honeymoon? Have you lost your mind, Levi? I came here to enjoy myself, not to be traumatized for the rest of my adult life!"

From that point on, I wanted to go home. I'd had my fill of Mexico. I swore that never again would I leave the U.S. unless God personally told me that I had to.

I refused to eat after that, convinced the food was not fit to eat, even at the resort, having only pizza, packaged corn nuts, or fresh fruit, and stuck to bottled water for the next two days because I felt certain that at least these things were all imported from the U.S.

Levi wanted a romantic dinner at the hotel restaurant. I wanted bottled water and corn nuts. I was determined that I was not going to die from food poisoning in Mexico, and Levi was not about to convince me to trust him. He had burned that bridge already.

"I do not care what you say to me. I am not putting that in my mouth. I will eat what I know is from America and that is it. If you don't like it, you can go straight to he**."

Levi became red-faced with fury. "Such stupidity. What more could I expect from someone from Ville Platte?" he said angrily.

When I ordered a pan pizza and the girl brought me a thin pizza, he chewed me out again when I demanded that she bring me what I had ordered.

"The girl didn't understand your Cajun accent, Jamie. It's not her fault; speak proper English, and maybe she will get you what you want."

Who was this rude and obnoxious man? I was appalled at the radical change in him. I had never seen him behave this way.

"Why are you treating me like this? Or has it totally escaped you that we are on our honeymoon?" I said to him furiously.

To which he retorted—quickly and crisply, "Jamie, the weeks we were dating—and you were demanding and even bossy—I thought it was cute at the time. But I also thought that you understood that once we were married, I was going to be the boss, and you were going to be submissive to me like the Bible says."

I could not believe the words I was hearing. Levi's statement did not go over well with me *at all*. I had no intention of changing my ways, ever. And the only submission I intended on doing was my life to the Lord, who was <u>not</u> Levi Guidry. I looked him squarely in his green eyes and, through clenched teeth, said, "So, you married me expecting me to change into someone else? Is that pretty much what I am hearing from you? Because if it is, you'd best know that I have no intention of changing who I am. I am quite happy with who I am—and unless God Himself changes me, you are quite stuck with this, Jamie. I will submit myself to the Lord, but I will not submit to any man, and that includes you!"

"Well then, you'll be in rebellion to God, and you'll be one miserable person," he retorted, "because it is God's will for a Christian wife to submit to her husband. You do believe the Word of God, don't you?"

I couldn't believe this was happening and, on my honeymoon, nonetheless. I was horrified and completely disillusioned.

What have I done? Mrs. Joy was so right. I must have lost my mind marrying this lunatic. Even Will had never spoken to me this way.

I just wanted to be back in the state and far, far from Cancun, Mexico. This honeymoon was amounting to a nightmare—from which I could not awake.

God, what have I done here? I gave up my relationship with the love of my life to marry this man who does not give a sh*** about me. And to say that God was in this marriage? How did I allow this to happen? Jamie, you disgust me!

It did not take long after our honeymoon for me to be haunted by the memory of Kerri's words on that pivotal, life-changing day: "When this doesn't work out, and it won't, **DO NOT CALL ME**.'"

And Mrs. Joy's words to me that she said with anger and pain in church the Sunday she learned that I was engaged to Levi: "Jamie, this man is not in love with you. He is simply looking for a wife. You just happen to be available. You will regret the day you marry him. Mark my words young, lady."

If only I had heeded what she had said. If only I had prayed about those words... how much pain I would have spared myself for many years to come.

The Unraveling...

Within a few short months, I began to fully comprehend just how awful my decision to marry Levi really was. The marriage was unraveling faster than I could put it back together. In our apartment in Eunice, about three blocks from Louisiana State

University, where I had enrolled to study, I began to sink into depression. One hot summer night, I woke up in a cold sweat after having had another nightmare, something that had been happening more frequently since the honeymoon. In all innocence and stupidity, I told Levi about it, hoping to get some comfort from him.

"I dreamed I married the wrong man, and a vision of Kerri's face came to my mind. In my dream, I was drowning and couldn't wake up. It scared me. Could you please pray for me so I can get back to sleep?"

To which Levi replied groggily, "Jamie, it is your body still trying to catch up to what the Spirit is doing in your life; of course, you didn't marry the wrong man. It was the Lord's will that we marry. You know that, and I know that. Now, go back to sleep."

Levi did not pray for me that night. In fact, he seldom prayed at all, from what I witnessed. The only time he prayed was when he wanted something from God. He prayed foxhole prayers of desperation and fear. But he never prayed simply to thank God or to praise Him.

The next morning, I woke up feeling exhausted from the lack of sleep. I couldn't help but think about the nightmare and wondered why Levi hadn't prayed with me. So, before he left for work, I approached him as he was drinking his coffee and asked him about it.

"Levi, why don't you ever pray for me or us? You want a submissive wife, but you refuse to submit to the God we are supposed to be serving together."

This went over like a lead balloon, as I should have known it would considering Levi's enormous ego. I have no idea what I expected from him, but it made Levi angry, and he replied defensively,

"Who do you think you are? My judge? I answer to God for what I do, not to you. You should remember that."

He then marched off to our bedroom, changed into his work clothes without speaking another word to me, and stormed out of the apartment.

Angry thoughts began swirling around in my head: *I know why you won't pray for me. Because you would first have to cast the devil himself out of you to pray for me. This man is no more a God-fearing man than one of Satan's archangels. In fact, the devil himself probably fears God more than he does.*

But I can tell you this much, Levi, you will burn in hell along with all the minions that helped you make this marriage happen. I may have been deceived, but I know that God is capable of making a way out, a way where there's no way.

Chapter 8

Too Many Changes

It was beginning to overwhelm me, and as time passed, I was beginning to lose Jamie. I was heartbroken and tormented at the same time as Lucrecia often reminded me of the horrible mistakes I had made in marrying Levi and losing Kerri. It was too much for me, both mentally and emotionally. This was NOT the life I had imagined as a married woman, a woman marrying the man God had chosen for her. How stupid of me. Just one more bad decision to add to the list. It was a growing list, to be certain, and I was regretting my mistakes more and more each day as one day blended into the next in my miserable married life with Levi ...

Levi and I had been married for only a few months when he decided he needed a career change. He had been the manager of a fast-food restaurant but lost his job when we relocated to Eunice so I could attend college at LSU-E. "I just cannot make it work here, Jamie," he told me one day. "I need to try a change. There's no opportunity here for me in Louisiana."

I wasn't excited about this news, but then it didn't surprise me. Levi was always looking for the next way to make a quick buck, no matter what I thought about his plans. What I wanted was of little or no concern to him, as I was quickly learning.

"Do what you have to do," I said to him. It was the most encouraging thing I could offer at the time. *It doesn't matter how far you run, Levi, you will never outrun yourself. No matter where you go, you will always be there!*

So, he went to work for a large trucking company as an over-the-road (OTR) driver, driving goods cross-country. I must admit it was nice to have him out of my hair. With him gone so much, I decided to move back in with my grandmother and mother since he was away so much. His small income just didn't pay enough to support me in an apartment, and besides, Grandmother was losing her battle with bone cancer. I needed to be near her.

It was excruciating to watch her withering away daily while experiencing such tormenting pain. She often moaned, grimaced, and even cussed at my Mother and me when we brought her medications and changed her feeding tube. In her morphine-induced paranoia, she was thinking that we were trying to poison her.

Watching her was an emotionally traumatizing experience that would haunt me for years to come.

I was an emotional mess. She had been my rock for years and, by far, my best friend.

From the hospital, I called Levi, devasted and still sobbing uncontrollably.

I wept bitterly from my broken heart and asked him to come be with me at the funeral. He was forced to quit his truck-driving job to come to the funeral. At least, that's what he led me to believe. *He never has money. Why is that?* I found myself asking. *I don't believe for a minute that he is repaying truck-driving school loans. Think of all the times, Jamie, when he hasn't been reachable. What was he doing? Where was he?* I was learning more, all the time, that he wasn't the most honest or forthcoming man on the planet by a long shot!

After the funeral, Levi took me to eat at the Pig Stand restaurant to get my mind off Grandmother and for a change of scenery. I was not prepared, however, for the topic of our conversation.

"I was offered a job in Colorado at a ski ranch. They want to hire us both. It's beautiful, right in the heart of the Rockies."

How could he ask me to move right after I buried my grandmother, knowing how broken up everyone is? Because he does not give a rat's a** about me or my family. Levi cares about Levi!

"I am not comfortable with moving, Levi. My family needs me here. You go. Maybe I'll go later."

And then—right there in the driveway of the Pig Stand restaurant—Levi dropped to his knees, grabbed my hands, and begged, "I am your family now. Please, please come with me. You are my wife. I need you. I need you with me."

'Yes, yes, I realize I am your wife. It's my duty to be with you. I married you. I committed myself to you before God. I will forever rue that day!"

But he had managed, once again, to appeal to my sense of obligation … and once again … I fell for it. I knew that I had made a vow before my God and although my heart was far from him, I still felt that I had to honor that promise.

So, off to Colorado, we went.

Colorado Is Frigid

Gunnison, Colorado, was a rude awakening that winter. I wasn't prepared for how bitter cold it was, and after meeting our new bosses, I was none too excited about them either. "Levi, if she can't handle it at forty degrees here," said Teela, one of the co-owners of the ranch, about me, "what's she going to do when the temperature is minus forty?" Levi and Shane, Teela's husband, and the other ranch owner laughed at this. Their humor was lost on me. Teela and Shane were dressed in short-sleeved shirts and long pants, hardly outfitted for a cold winter day.

I, on the other hand, wore a long-sleeved turtleneck sweater, a thick jacket, and thermal underwear under my thick jeans, and still, I was shivering. Re-locating from Louisiana, where I shivered at 70 degrees, was shaping up into a real nightmare.

The only silver lining was the beauty of the snow-covered Rockies — they looked as though God had sprinkled powdered sugar on them. The scenery was totally breathtaking. The white glitter, which had been generously dusted everywhere, reminded me that Jesus was there in all His majesty, despite the misery I was enduring having to live with Levi.

'Oh, my God! Two brothers from a different mother. I have never met two rude men so much alike!

'Shane, you too are rude, bossy, obnoxious, and outspoken.

'I sit in horror as I watch you run the ranch like a dictatorship in which we are all far beneath you. Even Teela, and your daughter, Maddy, are set far beneath you. You sicken me much the same way my very own husband does.'

Shane, who was arrogant, obnoxious, and demanding most days, seemed to enjoy making me feel like an indentured servant. He was constantly picking apart every job I did as though I was completely inept.

"Jamie, why didn't you pass the rag on the bathroom walls as I asked you to and when I asked you to? He continued, "I don't like having to repeat myself to the help. We've had this conversation before. I guess I didn't make myself clear the first time, so I am addressing it again."

Feeling immediately defensive because I knew that I had indeed done what he asked me to do, I replied in the same tone he had spoken to me,

"Shane, I have no idea what you're talking about. I did wipe the walls of the bathroom, and I did it right after you asked me to. They may not have been wiped according to your standards or even your personal liking, but they got wiped with a wet rag, and I used bathroom cleaner also and Teela saw me doing it herself. Ask your wife if you don't believe me. Which, by the way, I don't make it a habit of lying. I do have integrity. Whether you believe it or not" … I retorted back to Shane in the same direct, aggressively rude manner he had delivered his speech to me, like he was talking down to me.

"I don't much like you Jamie, but I like Levi and he is a good worker, so I guess you get a pass."

"Oh, joy, lucky for me!" I replied to Shane in utter disgust, as I walked out of the restaurant and back to our room in the lodge. The man made my blood boil. OOOOOhhhh, I could not stand even being near him and it was even worse when he and Levi both got together. I had to swallow hard to remain a Christian when I was with those two men.

I was stuck in a very unpleasant and uncomfortable situation, and I knew it. Teela was scared that Shane might leave her and Maddy, so she followed along with his every whim and submitted to him much like a doormat being used to wipe his feet on. It was sad to watch.

Colder Than Mountain Air!

As Levi and I walked home from the restaurant after supper one bitterly cold evening, he lectured me about how I should act more like Teela. "You should spend some time with her. Maybe she would rub off on you." He was colder than the Colorado air.

"Yeah ... well, Levi, maybe you should spend some time with Jesus; maybe He would rub off on you," I retorted. "Maybe, it would do you some good. And then maybe, I would be interested in talking about submitting to you." I think he got the hint. The conversation was taking him nowhere fast.

After a few months of a hard, cold winter in the Rocky Mountains, I became increasingly restless and annoyed by my surroundings and, even worse, the company. Even the splendor of the scenery began to fail me. "I hate the cold here, Levi, it's bitter cold … there's no tv. He**, there's no radio either, and the phone only works twenty-five percent of the time."

"Yes, Jamie, that's why I like it so much. Fewer people and less drama."

I was lonely there and missed my mom and Kay. But to Levi's way of thinking, they were something I needed to leave behind. As he would put it, they were my "relatives," not my family. He was my family.

But I had grown to despise Silver Stone Ranch almost as much as I despised my husband, and I wanted to go home!

I started praying for the Lord to make a way for me to leave the ranch, whether Levi was with me or not. Enough was enough. Shane was an intolerable, obnoxious boss and Teela was nothing more than his doormat. "Lord, please make a way for us to leave this ranch. I hate it here. I need less snow, less cold, and more people. Please help me, but in all things Lord, I pray for Your will to be done."

Yes, please help us to leave before I hurt one of these people here and have to go to jail for it. I'm not feeling the whole orange jumpsuit thing today, Lucrecia screamed in my head.

Months after my pleadings to the Lord, Shane and Teela had us over for supper at their cabin. I knew something was up because this was a rare event. We normally ate at the restaurant, and Levi, and I had to stay behind and clean the kitchen. This was different, and although I liked the change, I had to wonder what the change was about. I didn't trust Shane any further than I could throw him.

Shane was grilling ribeye steaks and fresh vegetables for us all. It smelled so good, despite my ill feelings for the chef. I had grown tired of eating country-fried steak with white gravy or spaghetti or even meatloaf. I wanted some real food. This was a welcomed change of pace.

As we settled down for supper at the table, Shane finally let us in on the manipulation scheme—oh, excuse me did I just write that? I mean, he proceeded to tell Levi and me about his financial problem he was hoping we could help him solve.

"It would benefit everyone. I will sell you my check recovery agency back in Ohio. I know that you could do it. You're smart enough, and I know we can trust you. What do you think?"

No! It will totally benefit you, Shane! I thought disgustedly. *The good Lord knows that you are not about to do something that would benefit someone else.*

Levi and Shane spent the next several hours at the supper table that night, talking about the business venture while Teela and I cleaned up and got Maddy ready for bed.

Levi was all for it and had made his mind up before he ever heard a word from me as to my feelings on the matter. According to Levi, if he wanted my opinion, he would give it to me.

Levi, why you gotta be so incredibly dumb? Hasn't this man shown his wickedness enough for you to see that he has no care or concern for his own family, much less two people he hardly knows at all?

Moving... Again!

So, we picked up and moved again... And again, I was not happy with Levi or his decision. I didn't trust Shane or Teela either, for that matter. I had a hard time believing they would sell us a thriving company when they barely knew either of us.

"Jamie, can't you just trust me?" Levi asked me when I questioned the whole thing.

No, I couldn't. He never listened to me, and neither did he respect my opinion as his wife, who just might have heard from God herself. Imagine that!

I must say that Cincinnati was clean and charming. It had green rolling hills, and the sun shone bright most days. The temperatures were nice, about sixty-five to seventy, which was a far cry from negative twenty-five in Colorado. The people were a bit strange, however, very reserved,, and almost paranoid.

I recall driving home one day and waving to a stranger (which was something we did regularly back home), and a few people responded by flipping me off. I laughed out loud at this.

Shortly after the move to Cincinnati, my mother called me in tears from Ville Platte. She no longer had a place to stay. She was being forced to move because the family had sold my grandmother's house. "She can live here with us, but she will have to work with us at the company," Levi finally agreed.

I didn't like the idea myself, but I didn't feel that I could let my mom live on the streets. My mother was destitute, and I knew it.

So, at least I had my mom there with me. *Yeah, she will be here. I'm not sure if whether that will be a blessing … or a curse!* I worried to myself.

Next, Levi's best friend, Tom, also moved in with us. I despised this man almost as much as Levi when he was in Levi's presence.

We worked eight to ten hours a day, making phone calls, threatening people, and collecting bad checks, which included me, Levi, my mom, and Tom. It was hard work and, no matter what kind of effort we made. Still, it wasn't enough; the business was not producing the amount of money needed to keep its five offices afloat.

"I told you we couldn't trust Shane," I lectured Levi. Why would he sell us a thriving business with no money down? He just wanted you to take the fall so he could skate free."

This angered Levi because he felt that he was going to make his millions with this company.

'Right! That's a good one there!' I thought to myself as I laughed at Levi and his utter stupidity.

Chapter 9

God, What are You Doing???

The Box in the Trash

It was about three months into 1992, just after my twenty-second birthday, when I began to feel nauseated and overly tired. I went home early one day — alone — and took a pregnancy test. After the results confirmed what I was afraid of, I put the kit back into the box and placed the box in the trash, covering it with the lid. Out of sight, out of mind, right?

When Levi got home later, I was quiet and had been crying. He noticed the box in the trash when he threw his soda away and walked over to me with it in his hand. "Hey, what's this?"

"What does it look like? It's a pregnancy test. I guess we are going to have a baby."

Levi made no reply. He, too, walked to the trash can, put the box in the trash, and then put the lid back over the trash can. Guess he was no more excited about this news than I was.

My mother was ecstatic, however. "I'm going to be a grandmother!"

It was a difficult time for me. I was emotionally conflicted. I didn't want to be pregnant, and I certainly didn't want to have Levi's child. But at the same time, I knew that a baby was a blessing from God. The trauma of the conflicting feelings of the fear of being a mother and the disdain of being pregnant for Levi left me deathly ill.

I lost weight and dropped down from a hundred-ten to eighty-five pounds within weeks of learning I was pregnant. This was a concern for my doctor as well as for me. I couldn't even listen to a food commercial without running to the bathroom to vomit. It was the worst time of my life.

Unfortunately, I hated my husband, and I wanted to be rid of him—but he was the father of my child, and I was stuck.

I grew more pregnant by the day while feeling more and more exhausted and emotional. After a while, I was not able to go to the office anymore. It was simply too much for me to have the responsibility of a high-risk pregnancy and the stress of working full-time at a check collection agency. Something had to give because my health was quickly diminishing.

Bedrest for you, Jamie!

About seven months into my pregnancy, Levi decided that we needed to get out and do something fun. We had been at each other's throats for weeks, and the stress of the pregnancy, as well as the business, was destroying what little we had left of our relationship. So, we packed our SUV and took a day trip. We ended up at a park in Cincinnati, where there was an underground cave. This seemed exciting.

I had never been in a cave before and didn't know what to expect. Once in the cave, which was damp, cold, and cramped, I quickly learned that I was not good with dark, tight spaces. I began to hyperventilate and had a panic attack—my legs felt like they were made of jelly, my heart was beating out of my chest, and I was struggling to breathe.

Levi acted quickly and walked me out of the cave and to the SUV to get some fresh air. But it was too late. I couldn't calm myself down and began feeling pains in my stomach. I had never been pregnant before, so I called Mom and explained to her what had happened. She told me to get to the hospital quickly, "Jamie, you probably pushed yourself too hard, and it sounds like you are in premature labor."

Within minutes we were flying down the highway, emergency flashers on, and I was drinking water and praying. The prayers helped me calm down, but neither the water nor the prayers were calming down the contractions. I was terrified that I was going to lose my baby.

Once we got to the hospital, I learned that I was dehydrated, and that had caused me to go into premature labor. The Emergency Room (ER) doctor gave me a shot, and it stopped the contractions and saved my pregnancy. "Young lady, I am placing you on bedrest from now until week thirty-six. Go home and drink plenty of liquids and take care of yourself!"

If I am to be very honest, I must admit that I was not a good patient. Staying in bed was hard for me, and even though I was scared, I craved chocolate terribly. I had no vehicle, and the nearest store was behind the apartment about half a block away, through a field, so I would walk across the field and buy Ding Dongs at the little convenience store there … having contractions … stopping to breathe through them along the way. Slow and easy. It's going to be okay. Breathe … Practice your *Lamaze*. Breathe Jamie.

'*Dumb a** — you are going to have this baby in the field all alone,"* Lucrecia would berate me, "*and it will be hours, maybe even days, before anyone finds you. After all, who would think to look in a field for a woman who is pregnant and is supposed to be on bed rest?'*

Levi caught me one day coming home from the convenience store and became furious. "How can you be so irresponsible? You could lose our baby. Are you out of your mind, Jamie?"

This didn't exactly stop me from being stupid, but it did slow me down.

I began asking Levi to keep the apartment stocked with chocolate (Ding Dongs, chocolate chip cookies, and Rocky Road ice cream) so I only had to walk to the kitchen. It was nearly impossible to convince myself to stay in bed, but I did at least have the sense to stay in the apartment and do very little in the way of physical labor.

No, I wasn't entirely out of my mind, not quite yet. But there were days that it felt that way. My emotions were often out of control, and Lord knows my ability to make good rational decisions was questionable. With Lucrecia in one ear and my mental and emotional health waning more daily, it made for quite a life experience. I was in no shape to become a mother, yet motherhood was in my very near future...

A few weeks later, at week thirty-seven, our little bundle was born about an hour past midnight. It was a quick yet painful labor as I refused medication. But the pain subsided as soon as I heard my baby girl's cry. Tabatha Ariel was born on September 8, 1992.

I was so proud of my little baby, but still, I was an anxious mother, and my emotions were all over the place. I wasn't a good mom to her in the beginning. I was terrified and couldn't stop crying. I cried for nothing, and I cried for everything. I don't know if I was more afraid of her or of me. I became increasingly upset as the weeks passed and suddenly felt the need to be near my family. I felt no sense of happiness ... or hope at all ... and I cried some more. I wanted to be both a good mommy and I wanted to run away simultaneously.

I thought that I was going crazy for a time. I had never felt so low in my life, and I couldn't snap out of it no matter what I tried. It just got worse. I chided myself. *Jamie, your child needs you to be well. Snap out of it you dreadful woman. How can you be so selfish at such a time? Again, Lucrecia berated me. She never stopped.*

But that didn't work.

Nothing worked, and things just continued to spiral downward. I needed help. Out of desperation, Levi decided to move back home to Louisiana.

Baby Number Two has been Announced

Shortly after settling again in Eunice, amongst Levi's "relatives," I again began to experience nausea and excessive tiredness. This was about three months after giving birth to Tabatha. Having been there before, I knew what that meant. I bought a test … and what do you know? I was expecting another baby.

Trust me when I say this was *not* good news. I had been thinking of leaving Levi for months but, of course, had no way of supporting myself and one child. *How do you think you'd be able to support two, Jamie?* I choked back tears and anger. *Not three months from having Tabatha, and I'm expecting again? Barefoot and pregnant, that is how he wants to keep me, and so far, he has his way.*

This pregnancy was no easier than the first. In fact, after about six

Weeks, I began having hard contractions. I put myself on bed rest until I could see my doctor and began drinking plenty of fluids.

My doctor examined me, and I learned that I had an "incompetent cervix" and was lucky that I had never had a miscarriage. So, from the doctor's office to the hospital, I went to have a suture put around my cervix to prevent further contracting.

Mom was at home with Tabatha, and, as usual, Levi was not available. He was out "working" and wasn't answering his phone. I often found this quite suspicious since he didn't have a full-time job. He always claimed to be either working or looking for work.

I went to the hospital alone and finally showed up later that evening in a pseudo-panic. "Baby, I am so sorry I wasn't there for you. I am here now ... Blah, blah, blah."

Give it a rest Levi; we all know you don't care about me; you were probably chasing some skirt, and that's why you didn't answer.

By this time in our marriage, I had no care or concern whether he was with me or not. The more he was away, the less I had to hear his never-ending tirades. "Your dishwater is not hot enough. The water needs to be steaming when you do the dishes. You never cook, and when you do, where is the vegetable?" And more, "Can you please stop her from crying? I am trying to take a nap?" And on and on it went.

His demands and complaints were never-ending as things grew increasingly ugly. So, I began to complain. "Just leave me alone. Don't touch me, and please, please, do not force me to have sex with you again. I hate crying myself to sleep afterward."

It was not two weeks after I had a stitch put around my cervix and was placed on bed rest that Levi decided we were moving to Florida. It was my job, of course, to pack up the entire three-bedroom house and have it ready within three days to move. My mother and sister, Kay, were furious and begged me to leave him. They were fearful I would lose the baby and tear the stitch, and the real possibility of bleeding to death because of that.

If only I had some sense about me, but I stubbornly obeyed him, as in obedience to God. Little did I know that my merciful God would not have expected me to do something that would put both my and my unborn child's life in danger. I'm not sure what God I thought I was serving at that time. I dogmatically responded to their pleas with, "I married the fool. I need to stay with him."

So, off to Florida, we went, with no job and no plan.

Chapter 10

The Storm is A-Brewing

St. Petersburg, Florida, was scorching hot and miserable. Levi put us on the second floor of a two-story apartment building and then left me alone most days to care for Tabatha while I was supposed to be on bed rest. Levi spent his time looking for bikinis — oh I meant a job, of course, I meant to say looking for a job — and one day, instead, came home with a brilliant idea.

"I know someone who has a bikini bar on the beach and the girls wear bikinis and thongs. He needs a partner. I am going to go half with him, and we will make a fortune." I threw my head back and laughed haughtily in disgust.

"Levi, I cannot believe that you have sunk so morally low. If you think I am going to stay home barefoot and pregnant looking like a beached whale while you gawk and drool over the bikini-clad bodies of Florida, you have truly lost your da** mind. It is not even debatable. Now get out of my face before I lose my sh** with you."

Levi's face became red and so did his ears, which usually meant he was mad or embarrassed. I didn't care which it was. He admitted that he should keep looking for work.

"Yeah, Levi, that is what you should do, continue to look," I said with sarcasm, rolling my eyes and shaking my head.

Days after that conversation, a storm began to brew in the Atlantic. The 1993 "Storm of the Century," as it became known, was heading right toward St. Petersburg. I was terrified when I saw its size and trajectory. The next day Levi told me he had decided to take a trip back to Louisiana (out of harm's way) to sell our restaurant equipment, since he had depleted our savings "looking for work." I later learned from my brother, Jo, that Levi had spent his time at the beach checking out the view and had bragged to Jo about it.

I was horrified at the thought of Levi leaving us there, the storm coming straight at us, and me alone with Tabatha. I begged him not to go but he ignored me. "I will only be gone five days at the most. I'll leave the Maxima here and take the truck. If you need, go to a shelter with Tabatha," was all he said.

Daddy, Please Come Get Us!

I watched the weather channel for two days in horror as the storm became increasingly dangerous, and after much internal turmoil, I finally called my dad to come and get us. I knew he was going to be upset with me because just as Mom and Kay had begged, he also *begged me* to stay put while Levi went on ahead to Florida.

"Daddy, I need you to come get us. He left for Louisiana, and that storm is heading right toward us. Can you please come get us?"

We were barely on speaking terms, but he knew I wouldn't have called him unless I was in need. So, he came.

Just before Daddy arrived in Florida, Levi got home. I stewed over what to do but finally decided it was best to tell him that Daddy was on the way and that I was leaving with Tabatha. "My daddy is coming to get us. I have had enough. It was senseless, irresponsible, and cruel of you to leave us here to face that storm alone. I don't deserve to be treated this way. If I had known this was who you were, I would *never* have married you."

Upon hearing this, Levi decided, in his deranged mind, that the right thing to do was to sleep on the loveseat in the living room that faced the front door with a loaded 9mm pistol beside him on the floor.

I tried to call Daddy to warn him, but he didn't answer.

I knew my dad, and that situation was a disaster in the making. Someone was going to get hurt, one way or the other, and it was a chance I was not willing to take. Lucrecia screamed at me inside my head, *"Now look at this, would you? This idiot is going to have to eat his gun or kill our Daddy. Now what you gon' do with this, Jamie?"*

Panicked, I begged Levi to give me his gun, but he steadfastly refused, telling me he had the right to protect himself in his own home. So, after dark, when Levi was sound asleep, I snuck outside and called 911.

I waited outside the apartment while they crept in as he slept, five of them in battle-ready uniforms and helmets, looking like they were ready to attack if need be—to disarm him. They took his gun and told him that he could have it back once my dad had left town.

Levi was in tears when I walked in and visibly shaking. As I had been for days, he was terrified. I can't say that I felt any sense of empathy for him. He had brought all of it upon himself as far as I was concerned.

Daddy arrived the next morning with a sheriff's officer. He had figured that I would tell Levi and that it could be a dangerous situation.

I left with no fight as the officer kept the peace, taking Tabatha with me and half the money made from the sale of the restaurant equipment. Again, he had it coming to him.

Good Riddance, Levi!

It felt so good to be rid of Levi. Although it was hard being a single mom, I was used to the responsibility since Levi was so seldom home anyway.

Feeling as though I wanted to make my home in Ville Platte, I asked Daddy for help again. I knew he had resources, and within a week, he had found a Housing and Urban Development (HUD) house for me and Tabatha. I was so relieved to have a home. It was partly furnished, and I used the money from the restaurant equipment to set up our little house. Within a month of being in Louisiana, I had managed to modestly finish furnishing our place.

I didn't have a vehicle, but I knew that, too would come eventually., There was a store about a block from me, and Taunte and Nonc lived about a half-mile away.

I felt certain that I could make a go of it. I had a house phone but did not share the number with Levi, so it was peaceful there, and no one bothered Tabatha or me. Mom even came and stayed with me often to give me a break and help with the bed rest.

But my peace didn't last too long.

Levi was at my doorstep within a month, begging me to take him back.

"Jamie, I am sorry. It will never happen again. Please, please, just give me one more chance. I need you and Tabatha. I need my family," he said, trying to grab my hand as I pulled away from him. "Won't you even just hold my hand? You've never been this cold before."

I refused for a long time. I truly despised him. But when Jonah was born on October 13, 1993, I had a change of heart. I felt that I needed to give it another try since he was the father of my two children. This infuriated my entire family and put a greater wedge between Daddy and me.

"You're going to take him back after he had to be disarmed in Florida?" my daddy said. "Are you out of your mind, Jamie? If you do take him back, you will never see a dime of inheritance from me. I have no use for that man. You can also find another place to live. He will not live under a roof that belongs to me."

"Daddy, I appreciate all you did for me, but you will not control me with your money. I have to do what I believe is right for me and my family." It was a long time before my dad spoke to me after that day. He was angry and he was hurt.

Looking back, I can't say as I blame him. That was a pretty low blow dealt to him. Although Daddy was clearly not my favorite person on the planet, he didn't deserve that.

And I don't know why on earth I thought things would ever be different after going back to Levi. Clearly, there was something very wrong with my decision-making abilities. But what?

Chapter 11

The Nightmare on the Ranch

One morning over coffee, back in Eunice, Levi and I were sitting at the table eating oatmeal and fighting again as we fed the kids. It was a rare morning when he actually helped me with them. I should have known that it was manipulation at its finest.

"Jamie, we need to talk. Just hear me out before you say anything, please ..."

What now, fruit cake?' He had become a bobblehead toy to me by now. (He would bobble his head and move his mouth, but nothing with any sense came out.)

"Jamie, I cannot make it here. Eunice, Louisiana is not where it's at for me—or us. No matter how hard I try, we cannot get ahead. There is no money to be made here. The economy is dead. I cannot see raising the kids here. There is no opportunity, and I want more for me and the kids and you."

Was it just me, or had I heard this song and dance before? I was not liking where the conversation appeared to be going

"We need to move. I have called Shane and Teela … Don't freak out on me … Just hear me out."

"They have agreed to pay us both a salary! … and we will have our own apartment on the ranch! … they really want us to move back! They need us. Shane seems to have really changed … and I believe that God is opening a door." He waited expectantly until my shock wore off and I was able to respond.

"Levi! *God* is opening a door? I just don't know … I need to pray about this … It scares the hell out of me, the thought of trusting Shane again. You know he really screwed us. You could have ended up in jail over the business he sold to us. Why should we trust him?"

"Jamie, I knew that would be your attitude. But, I truly believe he has changed. He apologized to me for the ordeal with the business he sold us. I just don't know if I can do it," I replied. "I don't know if I care to trust Shane again; I just don't know if my heart can stand being there again. He really hurt me deeply, the lies … the deception … I just don't know, Levi."

Nevertheless, within two months, we were back in Gunnison, Colorado, at the ranch in the Rocky Mountains with Shane and Teela.

Again, instead of listening to the still, small voice, I listened to other voices-mine, Levi's, and Lucrecia's. Oh my, the heartache I could have spared me and my two children had I listened to God instead.

Same Crap, Different Day

Now, you would think that after giving up my home in Louisiana to relocate with Levi—again—that he would have appreciated me and shown me at least some respect, right?

No! That was not the case. ... Not ... at ... all.

Levi and Shane were like two peas in a pod and the devil was right in the mix with them. Nothing had changed; Shane still disrespected me and expected me to submit myself to Levi, as Teela submitted herself to him. But I was having none of it and made sure they all knew it.

But the fact is, I knew it was my fault I was in that mess, and Lucrecia made sure to rub my nose in it. *"Don't complain, missy. You did it to yourself. How many people have to scream at you not to do something before you listen to them? Hardhead, go on, be stubborn but don't complain when things don't go the way you saw them going. You shoulda listened to the people! Those who actually cared about you! Idiot! You wanted to marry him and now you want to run away. You best stay put, or God's gonna get you!"*

I stayed in prayer over our marital issues day after brutal day. But then, out of nowhere, things began to change ... Levi and Shane began to get on one another's nerves, giving me a blessed reprieve. *Praise you, thank you, Jesus.*

Levi even actually admitted that perhaps I had been right about not leaving Louisiana. "Maybe you were right about moving back here, Jamie. I am beginning to see another side to Shane, one that I don't like too much."

But it was too late. We were in Colorado, and the damage had been done. Besides, if he thought he regretted it at this point, he would know regret shortly. It was coming for him.

I never replied to him directly. It was too late for regrets.

Jeremiah 8:10

One morning as I entered the restaurant before the breakfast crowd filtered in, I overheard Shane and Teela talking about someone named José. Apparently, they thought pretty highly of him, and he wanted to come back to the ranch. They noticed me listening and changed the subject as I walked into the room.

Being less than discreet and unusually curious, I said, "So, who is José?"

Teela looked at Shane and then back to me and said, "He used to live here. He is Hispanic and loves the Lord. He left about a year ago to return home to his family in Mexico. He just contacted us. He wants to come back."

"Hmmm, okay,"

That said, I was no longer interested in the conversation.

"You will meet him soon, Jamie," Teela said, again looking at Shane and then looking back to me.

Wondering what the weirdness was about ... I said, "Okay if you say so,"

Shane asked, "Would you have a problem with a Hispanic person living with us here?"

"Nope. If he is a good person, that's all I care about."

The next evening I went into town with Shane and Teela. I needed to get out a bit, and this was my chance. It was precious seldom I was able to leave the ranch at all, much less without the kids. Levi had agreed to watch them, so I was altogether only too happy to leave.

Shane and Teela stopped by José's place on the way back home and I met him. He was a Mexican with jet-black, permed hair. He had a good sense of humor and was easy to talk to. They invited him to return to the ranch, and he accepted.

"What did you think of José?" Shane asked me on the way home.

"He seems nice. I don't know what else to say. Seems to be funny."

Shortly after, José moved back to the ranch. He was, indeed, very funny and full of stories and jokes. He brought a lot of laughter with him to the ranch, and that was refreshing. I think that even Levi liked him. He appeared to have a relationship with God, and that was also a relief after the psycho-Christians I had been living around for the last few months.

One day when I was cleaning the restaurant, Shane and Teela approached me. The somber look on their faces scared me. "What is it? Are the kids okay?"

"Yes, everyone is okay, but we need to have a serious talk with you. Can we all sit for a little bit? The clean up can wait a while."

Shane seemed so serious. Teela too, for that matter. I soon understood.

"I have been praying for you, and I believe God has given me a word for your life," Shane began, opening his Bible and reading from Jeremiah, "Therefore, I will give their wives to other men and their fields to new owners. From the least to the greatest, all are greedy for gain; prophets and priests alike, all practice deceit."

"Jamie, this is from Jeremiah 8:10," said Shane. "You see, God has heard your urgent prayers. He is replacing Levi. That is why José has returned to the ranch. We believe it is God's will for you to be with José. He has seen the greed and deceit of Levi. He is not pleased. José is a Godly man, and we believe that God has spoken this to us."

Needless to say, I was shocked and began to cry. I had been praying for God to deliver me from Levi and his ugly ways. I just didn't think God had heard me. A huge feeling of relief began to wash over me.

Once I was able to gather myself enough to speak, I finally asked, "What about Levi?"

"He will be sent home to Louisiana," said Shane. "He is not worthy of you. Pray about it, Jamie. We know God will confirm this to you as He has to José."

Did God really hear my prayers? Is this the miracle I have been praying for?

Is This the Will of God?

I prayed hard that night and asked for confirmation from the Lord in terms that I could understand. I needed to know that this was God's will. But inside my head, I was having all kinds of conflicting thoughts.

What the hell is wrong with you, Jamie??? I just have to wonder when I think about this happening in my life. What the hell am I thinking???'

The next morning, I went down to the restaurant with the kids taking notice of the beauty of the snow-dusted mountains. It was almost surreal. The snow was like sparkling diamonds when the sun hit it. Truly it was the work of the Lord's hand as He displayed his majestic works in all His splendor. As I looked at the scene before me, it was obvious that God was here with me. I knew it. I needed to see José. I needed to talk to him.

"José, Shane, and Teela told me about the Word from the Lord. What do you feel? I am so scared of not doing the will of the Lord. I need to hear from you. I trust you hear from God," I said to him. Even as I was speaking the words, I couldn't believe they were coming out of my mouth. *Where is that girl of nineteen who heard from God for herself?* I thought incredulously. *Where has she gone?* ·

"Jamie, I have prayed about it. I know that it is hard to believe, but I, too, feel that God has spoken. Levi is on his way out. He does not appreciate what God has given to him. He is being replaced. I only hope that I can make you a good husband and make you happy. I am willing to tell Levi if you are scared to tell him yourself."

Again, I was stunned. I was talking to the man my Heavenly Father had supposedly chosen to replace Levi. He was a Godly man, surely, he was... I was surprised at how I was being led so easily down this path, and all because I thought it was God's will.

That afternoon, Shane and José spoke to Levi, and he was escorted off of the ranch. I was both sad for Levi and relieved at the same time. He took the bus home and never questioned Shane, José, or me about my decision to leave him for another man. It was so unlike him not to fight. Perhaps he was as relieved as I was?

Or perhaps something else was going on that no one would ever suspect. Something entirely unrelated to my relationship with Levi. I would always wonder, looking back. Something just didn't add up. But what?

And even more importantly, what did all of this say about Jamie? How did I allow myself to get into such a mess as to marry a man I hardly knew while still in love with someone else? Then to leave him for a man I just met because GOD said so, according to two people I never liked or trusted from the first day I met them? What was I thinking? Where was my ability to think critically or rationally? Where had Jamie gone and how could I get her back again?

Chapter 12

My Second "God-Chosen" Husband

What can you be thinking, Jamie?

I pushed any warning thoughts out of my head about my plan to leave Levi and start a life with José, a man I barely knew.

"Hmmm, why does this sound so familiar, Jamie?" I heard Lucrecia scream at me. *"Really, Jamie, really? How can you be so stupid? Didn't you leave Kerri for a man you hardly knew?"*

But I had been so traumatized and so mistreated living with Levi that I didn't care how he got out of my life, even if it meant starting a new one with a total stranger that had been supposedly given to me by God.

So, before the end of the week, I had moved José in with me and the kids. If it was God's will, I didn't see any reason to prolong our becoming a family. I was ready to be happy, and this was my time; this was our time!

But Shane and Teela did not approve —they felt I needed to wait for the divorce from Levi and to be married to José before living with him. This was the one thing they said to me that was absolutely right. But I insisted that if God had replaced Levi with José, it was done.

Shane wasn't having any of it. He made it clear that I was going to follow his plan for the way things would go down, and not my own, as he and Teela were planning to sell the ranch and work on a boat, and José and I were going to be coming along.

"You see where God is leading us, right?" he said. "We need to pour our lives into serving God. Wouldn't you agree that we would be safer from being tainted by the world if we were alone, like on a ship … on the ocean? Just us and God?"

"*What?* Shane, I am not going on a ship with you or anyone else for that matter. It ain't happenin'."

He was emphatic. "Jamie, you will either sell José on the idea, or y'all can leave the ranch because we will be selling it and boarding a ship within the next three months."

Two weeks later, José was heading north, and I was heading south. He had a friend in Oregon who was doing construction and agreed to hire him. And I, again, reached out to Daddy.

"Can you come get me? I am leaving the ranch with the kids." He didn't seem too surprised by my call and never asked about Levi.

Daddy picked us up at the airport, but he was not happy about it. I had no place to stay, so I had to live with him and his new wife, Mrs. D. It was very awkward, to say the least. I felt like such a burden. So, the next morning I was on the phone asking Taunte and Nonc if we could live with them for a short time, me and the kids. I left a note explaining that since Taunte and Nonc's house was closer to town, it would be easier to find a job and a ride living at their house.

Meanwhile, José was sending me money from Oregon every week, as he had promised. He even sent me clothes to wear at the job I was blessed to get, working as a bank teller. Within a month, I had saved up enough to move into a trailer of my own, a three-bedroom right down the road from Taunte and Nonc and only about five miles from the bank where I worked.

It was time for mom and José to meet when José moved in with me, mom and, the kids once I had the trailer. That went over like a lead balloon. Mom and José were like two opposite ends of a magnet from day one. José didn't like her much or Ville Platte, either. He felt he was treated with prejudice and couldn't find work anywhere. He was very discouraged. I should have known that something was up when José informed me that I was too hard on my kids and needed some time away from them.

The idea was abhorrent to me. But I was so exhausted from the past dealing with Levi and now the fighting between José and Mom that I was emotionally worn thin. Plus, Levi had always told me I was too rough on the kids, so when José began with the same criticism, I heard Levi's voice and it scared me.

I didn't see it then but telling me I needed to leave my kids was his way of getting out of Ville Platte. Because I trusted him and his motives, he managed to convince me to leave my responsibilities behind." Jamie, you have been through enough, constantly fighting with Levi and having no time for yourself. Let Levi take the kids for a little while, and let's get out of here. We can travel for a while, and then, when you are stronger, you can take the kids back. You're stressed, and you're going to end up hurting one of them, and then you will never forgive yourself."

At first, I resisted, but he didn't give up.

"Jamie, your kids are better off without you right now. You are tired, and you need a break. Levi is their daddy. They are his responsibility, too, not just yours. You are not giving them away. You are just asking for a break and time to rest."

I was scared to death of harming my children and didn't have the strength to fight. Finally, I agreed to go for a short time. I told Levi to come and get the kids, saying, "I will be back, and at that time, I will want them back."

Levi was angry and immediately filed abandonment charges against me, and I lost custody of the kids to him. I was devastated. I hadn't pictured things turning out that way in my wildest dreams.

God, Where Are You?

José and I lived out of a tent in the Kamprgronds of America (KOA) campground just outside of Alexandria, Louisiana, for about six weeks to take a break from the responsibilities of civilization and adult life. We talked and walked and prayed all day, which speaks volumes about just how deceived I was at that time.

Hmmm, not divorced from Levi and not married to José... isn't that adultery, Jamie? I would wonder to myself. *But, I was given to José by the Lord, under the authority of the Word in Jeremiah 8:10. That isn't adulterous.*

I had convinced myself that I was justified. In my deluded state of mind, I never felt one iota of guilt about leaving my children or being in a relationship with José because I reasoned, I was closer to God than I had been in years. Yes, even in my delusion, God still took care of me and answered my prayers. He provided me with a job, my home, and the support of my loving family. That's the love of our Father!

After weeks of living on sandwiches and water in the KOA campground, the money we had saved ran out, and we were without a plan. Although I praised God for His goodness, there were times I wondered if God had turned His back on me and was angry with me because I had given my kids to Levi. But José refused to believe we had made a mistake. "He is just testing our faith. We have to push on."

I was in prayer over the lack of finances and saw the face of an ex-employee from our days in Ohio in my mind's eye. In desperation, I contacted her and begged for help. I was shocked that she agreed to assist me. We were never close, and I had been ugly to her. I felt her willingness was an answer from God. What else could explain her kindness? She bought us bus tickets, and within a week, we were back in Ohio.

I began to feel depressed and homesick and missed my kids so badly. I literally ached all the way into my bones when I thought of them. I decided then that I needed to return home. Dena had urged me to go back: "You need to be with Levi and your kids. You were deceived at the ranch. This is not God's will to be away from your family. Let me call Levi for you. He needs to know what you've been through. Whether he likes it or not, he brought you to that ranch. He is partially responsible for what took place there."

After many months of deception, I was ready to admit it had all been a farce—that the enemy was trying to destroy my family and my testimony. I had been deceived, and I believe that Shane, Teela, and José had been deceived. Now I was ready to fight to get my family back. "Please help me. I feel so lost," I told Dena, "Thank you for what you have done."

That night she contacted Levi for me and explained to him that I was deceived at the ranch and was ready to return home. Levi hadn't known the whole story, so she filled him in. He was furious.

The next morning, she explained it all to me, ending with, "Levi is willing to give your marriage another try."

The next evening I told José that I was returning home to Levi. I broke it to him as gently as I could. He did not take it well. This huge beast of a man became furious, revealing the psycho side of himself to me, which he had warned me of previously. He picked me up by my throat, dangled me like a rag doll with my feet off the ground, and then threw me onto the paved blacktop road. As I lay there looking at him in utter fear, wide-eyed and pale, he caught his head with his hands and said, "You stupid little bi***, are you trying to make me kill you?" The insane look in his eyes terrified me. He then took off running down the road.

I never spoke to José again.

I could not believe what I had done to myself, leaving my kids and yoking myself to this crazy man. And to top it all off, Lucrecia's voice was back, roaring her thunderous accusations against me. *"I have to say, Jamie, this is a royal screw-up. First, you throw Levi off the ranch, then you take another man in, then you dump the other man, and now you want to return to Levi? Girl, you are certainly a piece of work. And what were you thinking, being with that dude? He was absolutely insane, and you are lucky he didn't kill your dumb a**.*

"You need to get your sh** together, girl! You are a pathetic excuse for a human being at this point. You best get ready to grovel. You know Levi is going to run you through hell and back over this one! You have really dug a hole for yourself this time!"

Reunited

Levi was furious with Shane, Teela, and José, but also told me that he felt as though he shared part of the blame for taking us back there. "Jamie, we can make this work. I feel so humiliated that I ever took you back there. I certainly shoulder my share of the blame for what took place. Please forgive me for what you went through at their hands."

It was a start. This was the first time Levi had apologized to me with any kind of sincerity. I believed that God was at work.

I returned home to Levi and the kids three days later on a Greyhound bus. I wish I could say that it was a glorious reunion, but I would be lying.

Although Levi apologized to me over the telephone when I was in Cincinnati, it was a different story once I got home to him and the kids. He took no responsibility and treated me like someone who had simply decided to cheat on him. My apologies fell on deaf ears. "But where," I asked, "is the Levi who apologized just days ago over the phone? Where did he go?" Levi avoided those questions altogether. But I knew that I had gotten my point across. I had been through enough, and I was going to speak my mind whether he liked it or not.

But I was still scared to death of him leaving and taking the kids since he had full custody, so I gave in to him a lot even though we fought. Oh, how we fought … and then some. Again, I prayed for our marriage, our family, and strength to either endure the pain … or leave for good.

"I am so sick of my pathetic life. I have trusted so many people only to be used, deceived, and passed around from person to person like a dirty hand rag. I'm at the end of my rope here! Something has to give. I can't deal with this cold man or his negative, manipulative ways. He is one person in front of his church friend and another person at home."

All I could do was pray … and pray I did.

Chapter 13

Slow Down, Jamie!

Just as sure as a leopard cannot change its spots, Levi had not changed one bit while I was away. He had spent "countless hours in church, praying," and yet, it had done nothing to draw him any closer to God. I was so disillusioned by this realization after having been home for only a few months. Once the newness of my return wore off, Levi began his degrading tirades once again.

"Can you cook a decent meal for supper? I am tired of gumbo and soups. I want rice, gravy, and a vegetable … And, when you clean the kitchen after cooking, you need to use something like Clorox in your hot water. It helps to kill germs. And the water needs to be steaming hot, not lukewarm."

"If you don't shut up, I am going to put you in a blender and cook your rotten a** and feed you to the neighbor's pit bulls," Lucrecia would say inside my head.

I must have been out of my mind to marry this man. I would argue with myself. *I just don't know what was wrong with me. So many bad choices, and things just go from bad to worse no matter how hard I try. My heart is in the right place, but my decision-maker is broken!*

I fought with these kinds of thoughts regularly. I just knew there was something wrong with me. I knew it, and I could feel it. I just couldn't get it right, no matter how hard I tried. And to top it all off, I had managed to let myself get pregnant again by this disgusting man.

But despite all that, Gabrielle Nicole became my tiny blessing on January 26, 1996. She was beautiful, and I was glad to be a mommy again. Her birth was a bright spot in my dark world. But it did not fix the marital problems. Still, we disagreed, and still, Levi was displeased with his wife, who was at this point feeling like she was going crazy.

It was then that "Dr. Levi" (didn't know he had a medical degree, did ya?) made his official "diagnosis" of me, the one that would come back to haunt me at Carson City General Hospital, "You are bipolar, no doubt about it. You were abused and neglected in your childhood, and that's why you're crazy."

The D.I.V.O.R.C.E.

I spent a lot of time with my three kids while Levi was out and about, either looking for work or avoiding it, perhaps both. He hated work. He was a student at Louisiana State University at Eunice at this time, studying to become a paramedic or a nurse … my memory fails me. He was always coming up with new ways to run away from himself and his situation. At one point, he thought it would be a good idea to move to the Caribbean to study medicine outside the U.S., then come back to the U.S. with a medical degree. "It would save me so much time and money. What do you say?"

Of course, I said no.

I was sick of his hair-brained schemes. He was always looking for a way to make a quick buck, another great idea that was a sure thing. Yet, still, I had to pray for someone to bless us with money to pay our water or light bill.

It was quickly becoming apparent that I was going to need the ability to support my family one day. One of us needed to use our brains and get a real education.

Within a few weeks, I was awarded financial aid to return to school, including student loans and a Pell Grant. I was ecstatic. With this, I was going to have access to freedom — freedom from Levi and freedom from the ever-present fear of moving again. My children and I needed stability, and I was going to provide that for us no matter how hard I had to work. We deserved it.

Levi didn't take the news about my award letter very well — his face became pale — he could see the writing on the wall and knew exactly where this conversation was going...

"The kids and I are moving to Ville Platte at the end of the month. You can come, or you can stay, but we're moving. I need to be near my family so I can have help with the kids while I'm in school."

Levi's face went from pale to red as he turned on me in anger.

"Jamie, I am not moving to Ville Platte. I have nothing for that town. If you move there, it will be without me. We will be parting our ways. Are you sure that's what you want?"

"I am moving to Ville Platte," I replied calmly. "If you want to part ways over that, that's your choice. I am fine with that."

As I packed us up, I had mixed emotions. I was excited to get on with my life, but I also felt lost. I hadn't married Levi with the intention of ever divorcing him, but I knew that the children and I couldn't continue the way we were.

Kay and Jo helped move into a house just outside Ville Platte. Levi stayed behind as he said he would. Levi provided little in the way of support but showed up often in Tommy Hilfiger or Ralph Lauren clothes, complaining that he had no money to support me and the kids if we weren't going to all live together. He was trying his best to punish me for my choice to separate. More than once, I thought about how I would like to feed him his shoes or plant my foot firmly in his rear end for his stinginess.

Only a Shadow of My Former Self

The move to Ville Platte was so much harder than I anticipated. I began to feel like there was nothing left of my former self. Suddenly I recalled an argument I had with Daddy on his back porch about three years earlier. "Jamie, you are only a shadow of the person you used to be," he had told me. This made me angry, but he had been right. I truly had lost sight of who Jamie was, and now I felt like nothing more than a shadow of the real me. … I had become so consumed with trying to change myself to please Levi and prevent us from fighting that I didn't even know who I was anymore. Maybe I was more Lucrecia than Jamie, I wondered.

Maybe I am more Lucrecia than Jamie now; I would sometimes wonder.

By day's end, I was beaten and had little energy to apply to homework. My grades (normally A's) were suffering, and I was getting B's and C's. It was all I could muster.

Struggling to pay the bills, go to school, and keep my grades up so I could keep my financial aid was tough. But honestly, the greatest challenge was trying to find Jamie again. I had no idea who she was anymore and was so disappointed with who I had become. I second-guessed every decision. Being in a relationship with a man who had berated and belittled everything I did had taken its toll and done a number on my self-confidence despite how hard I had fought to maintain my identity. I hadn't realized how much of Jamie I had lost until now.

Often I had to give myself pep talks: *Jamie, girl, you gotta get it together. These kids need you. They need their mom to lead and guide them. You gotta do this thing!* I fought to endure each day without drinking or cussing.

I was grateful for those who supported me, like my then-best friend, Deb, a grade school pal. "If anyone knows that you can do this, it's me," she said one day. "Yes, I know it's hard, but you've got this, Jamie." It was so nice to spend time together again as we had been friends all through high school, but Levi had seen to it that our friendship had died along with Jamie during our marriage, so I was very happy to have her back in my life again.

Other people, whom I had counted on for help so much in the past, decided I'd made a mistake leaving Levi and refused to help me. Taunte and Nonc were among them. One day, when I asked them to babysit, they refused, saying, "You know he took you back after you went with that Mexican. He must have some good in him. You need to be with your husband. Those kids need their daddy." I left their place feeling so defeated.

The separation was hardest on my kids. Levi seldom saw them because he had "no one to watch them" so he could work. I told him over and over, "They need to spend time with you too. Come and get them, at least for the weekend. I didn't make these kids alone. They are your responsibility too!"

Finally, after a few months of fighting with him, I found an attorney and filed for divorce.

Can I Take You to Dinner?

One day after work and school, I received a phone call from a friend of Levi's. I was shocked to hear from him. It was Tom. He called to tell me he was in town because his mom had passed.

He wanted to see me, which surprised me. "Tom, Levi and I are separated now and going through a divorce. Are you sure it is *me* you want to see?"

Though they had been friends, Levi and Tom hadn't spoken in years due to a disagreement over the business in Cincinnati. I had always felt that Levi did to Tom what Shane had done to us, and I had confronted Levi about it.

"Yes, Jamie, I am certain it is you I want to see. Could I take you out to eat while I am in town?"

I had nothing to lose at this point, and I was curious as to what Tom wanted with me, so I found a sitter and agreed to meet him.

Later that week, Tom showed up with flowers and candy. I was pleasantly surprised. I had not been given flowers from a man in a long while.

We went to Prejean's Seafood, which I heard was a nice place both to eat and to listen to good Cajun music. I was not disappointed in either.

Tom had tried to grab my hand on the way inside, which took me by surprise. I pulled away from him.

"You don't want to hold my hand?"

"Tom, I am confused, really. Can you tell me what this is about?"

"Jamie, I have been wanting to tell you something for years, but you were a married woman, *and* you were married to my then-best friend. The truth is, I have been in love with you since the first day we met. I was so jealous of Levi because I wanted you." Continuing, he said, "You are such a beautiful person, and it was so hard for me to sit and watch the way Levi treated you. I tried to tell him he should be better to you, but he was convinced that he was within his rights. So, when I heard you had filed for divorce, I prayed God would see fit to open your heart to give me a chance."

I was stunned, to say the least. "Tom, I don't know what to say. I thought you hated me. I am shocked. You're going to have to give me a minute to absorb this."

We ate and had a great time reminiscing about Cincinnati. I sat there thinking about how very judgmental I had been of Tom because I felt that he drank too much and was way too irresponsible with his numerous girlfriends. I apologized to him then for my judgmental attitude towards him.

"Tom, I was very hard on you in Cincinnati. I have grown up since then. I am so sorry."

"Jamie, that's in the past, and in many ways you were right. The Lord had to deal with me about my drinking and partying. I, too, have grown up since then. No need to apologize. Let's forget about it."

I invited Tom in when we pulled up to my little house after dinner. We stood right in front of the space heater in my tiny living room just to keep warm and talked. As he was getting ready to leave, he leaned down and kissed me. Again, I was taken by surprise.

What was even more surprising to me was that I didn't shy away from his kiss, and it woke up emotions that had been dormant for years. I realized then that I had feelings for Tom too. I went to bed smiling that night, which hadn't happened in a very long time.

Chapter 14

Another Faux Pas

Tom began calling me long distance, daily. Once I put the kids to bed, we'd talk for hours. It was an expensive vice and Tom soon had phone bills upwards of a thousand dollars a month. "Jamie, I am going to buy you a cell phone," he told me one day. "I know you can't afford it, but I can't afford to pay thousands a month in long distance phone bills."

It was hard maintaining a long distance relationship. Tom complained because I seldom stayed home and often forgot to take the cell phone with me. Truth be known, I hated it and felt like I was on a leash. I didn't appreciate the feeling of being controlled, but I did understand that Tom missed me and wanted to know that I was okay since I lived alone with the kids. Sometimes this reminded me of Levi, who always wanted to know my every move. It rubbed my independent nature the wrong way. But I agreed to stay in touch with him better using the cell phone. "I will work on my need for independence!" I assured him, "Thanks for worrying about me and the kids."

With time, Tom and I got closer and closer. I learned to trust him as he said and did all the right things, it seemed, But I did choose to overlook some behavior that should have made me think twice.

"Jamie, you should have seen this! I was at a bar, and this girl was literally stripping on a table. I couldn't believe it!"

"Tom, you mean you didn't leave when she did that? How would you have felt if I would have stayed and watched some man strip in a bar?" I asked him in disgust.

Tom had a different set of standards for him than for me. I saw that in retrospect, but not at the time we were dating. In his mind, I needed to be at home with the kids doing schoolwork, but it was fine for him to go to the bars and drink until all hours in the morning. This should have been a red flag. Tom was supposed to be a follower of Christ and setting an example for my children.

"Jamie, you have your kids and your family around you. I have no one. That's why I go to the bar. It's lonely being home alone all the time. Please try to understand where I am coming from."

Tom liked his Long Island Iced Tea—a lot. This concerned me because I was not and never had been much of a drinker. Tom gave the same argument about his drinking habit.

"Jamie, I just get lonely, and drinking helps me cope. Please don't hold it against me. You just don't understand how hard it is to be all alone. I need a distraction, and my job is so stressful. It helps me to relax."

I had started to pray about the situation. "Lord, please help me make a good choice where Tom is concerned. I don't want to make another mistake. I really care for him, I believe I even love him, but I am so scared to trust my feelings at this point. I have made so many mistakes in the past, and I have three kids to think about now. It's not just about me anymore. Please protect me and my kids from any plans of the enemy to destroy us. If Tom is not the man for me, please let me know."

I told Tom how much his drinking scared me. "Jamie, the Lord healed me of that years ago. I have a handle on my drinking now," he told me. "I can stop and walk away. I am asking you to please trust me. I love you and the kids. I would never do anything to hurt any of you. You have to believe that."

Tom was good to me while we were dating, and I believe it was that "goodness" that persuaded me to overlook the red flags. He made good money and had no problems spending it. We did plenty of that while we were long distance dating. Each time I went to visit Tom, he had an adventurous trip planned, and we thoroughly enjoyed one another's company.

He took me to Yosemite and enjoyed the Pacific Ocean as we traveled Highway One along the coast of California. We went to Napa Valley and visited the various wineries. He took me to San Francisco to see Little China Town and Pier 39. Tom spared no expense. We slept in ritzy hotels and ate in nice restaurants. It was all amazing!

These trips were unbelievably lavish. Coming from a seven-year marriage in which my financial situation was devoid of any kind of security, this relationship with Tom and the mini-vacations were impressive and unexpected allurements. As I look back now, I see where I mistook those trips as Tom's way of showing his love for me.

But I was too easily enamored by what appeared at first glance to be Tom's generosity and desire to bless me. If I had prayed more, I might have seen through this tactic. But the truth is I prayed with my eyes shut tightly with my hands over my ears. I simply did not want to be alone, and Tom showed interest in me. All it took was for him to show an interest while throwing money my way and I was hooked.

I Know This Feeling

It must have been mid-March when I began to notice that I was gaining weight and was constantly hungry. I knew what this meant—no boxed test necessary—and immediately made an appointment with my doctor. He confirmed what I had been suspecting- baby number four was on the way.

I laughed at this as I remembered a conversation with Tabatha a few months earlier. "Mom, I want a baby brother, and we will name him Benjamin." It would appear that the Lord had heard her request. (Now to see if it was a boy or a girl.) But I already knew in my heart that baby Benjamin was on his way.

That night I had a huge surprise for Tom when he made his nightly call to me.

"Tom, I have something to tell you. I would have preferred to tell you in person, but I don't want to wait. Remember when Tabatha said that she wanted a baby brother named Benjamin? Well, it appears that God heard her request. We are going to have a baby in December!!"

"What??? Are you serious? You're pregnant? Jamie, I am beside myself. I have been praying for a son. I just know that God is going to bless me with a son. Praise the Lord!"

It certainly wasn't ideal circumstances. We weren't married, and I had to worry about the possibility of a premature labor so without telling anyone, I had a suture put around my cervix. Tom wasn't happy that I had chosen not to tell my family and done this alone, but it had to be done.

As excited as Tom was about the pregnancy, I realized there were some issues of trust between us. While I had been faithful to him, it appeared that he wondered about that.

One afternoon after work Tom called me and began our conversation with a weird hesitation in his voice. "Jamie, I have had several of my friends here ask me if I was sure that the baby is mine. But I told them that I trust you."

This statement coming from the man who sat at a bar and watched girls strip in front of him did not sit well with me, to put it mildly.

"Tom, if you trust me, why did you even bother to tell me that? Are you worried? I know I am certain of who this baby belongs to, but if you're not, take a paternity test. That's all I can tell you.

"No, Jamie, that won't be necessary. I know that I can trust you, and that is what I have told my friends."

But it was too late. He had basically accused me of sleeping with other men. That night I cried myself to sleep. It seemed so unfair that all I did was attend school, work, and raise three children while Tom went to the bar every weekend. Yet, I was the one who was not to be trusted.

That night I prayed. *"Lord, please deal with Tom. That was so uncalled for. I don't deserve to be questioned about my faithfulness. He was wrong for that."*

God was so faithful. Over and again, I took my issues to Him, and Tom would come back with an apology. The next afternoon Tom called me and apologized for questioning my faithfulness to him: "Jamie, I just get scared. You are young and beautiful, and I am old, fat, and ugly. It's hard to believe that I have such a beautiful and intelligent girl who wants to be with me. But it's no excuse for my behavior. Please forgive me."

I thanked him for apologizing, it meant a lot to me. It was moments such as those that made me feel safe with him. He was human and made mistakes, but he owned them and apologized when he was wrong.

He also heard from God. That was important to me. I had been with a man who proclaimed to know God, but who had shown little evidence of it. This man seemed to be different.

As it became more obvious that I was carrying Tom's baby Levi was beside himself with rage. To hear him tell it, I had stolen his best friend and done so just to spite him.

As we prepared to move out to Carson City, Nevada to be with Tom, Levi became more and more agitated. Levi's main concern was having the children to use to control me. He didn't want me taking our children out of state. But as far as I was concerned, I was their mother and they needed to be with me. Plus, Levi was alone and had no one to really help him. Jamie, I will fight you to the end of this," he threatened. But by this time, I didn't care much about Levi's threats. He would just have to suck it up because I was going… and the kids were coming with me!

By this time, nearing the end of summer 1997, I was happy with my life. The divorce was finalized, I was awarded custody of the children, and Tom and I were married a few days later in Sand Harbor, Lake Tahoe, Nevada.

It was time to begin the next chapter of my life and I looked forward to putting the past behind me.

Chapter 15

Hello Nevada!

*L*ife was about to change, not only for myself but for my children as well. We were leaving what we always knew (Louisiana) behind and embarking on a new and exciting future. How I looked forward to putting the awful memories of the past behind us and healing from it…Although I had not been formally diagnosed with a mental illness up to this point in my life, I knew that I had struggled with depression, especially after the births of my three children. I was certain that this one was going to be different. Things were looking up…

Benjamin's birth was fast approaching, and though we had just been married, there was no time for a honeymoon. I had to prepare for the kids to come up from Louisiana as well as the birth of Benjamin … I was anxious to get my home ready for the birth. I was "nesting," as Tom called it.

But in all this preparation, things did not go as smoothly as I would have liked. Tom was much more inclined to let me do all the work and chores while he did a lot of observing and complaining.

"Jamie, I know that you are 'nesting,' but I am not used to doing much after work. I have a stressful job, and it seems that you want me to work all day and then come home and work some more. I must say, I don't like that."

"Tom, I am pregnant for Christ's sake" I replied. I can't do all this by myself. We need to move into a bigger apartment. These two bedrooms are too small for all of us. We have a short time before the baby is here and I want everything ready for him. Why can't you understand that I need your help?"

Thankfully, Tom's church friends came to the rescue. I found a three-bedroom apartment, and they all came over and helped us pack and move. I was so grateful to each of them for their kindness.

I noticed a pattern was forming with Tom that I was not liking and had not seen in him up until this point. He did a lot of pointing and directing, but not a lot of actually doing anything else. One thing I did not like was a man who was willing to allow others to assume his responsibilities. I had that before with Levi, and I was not going to have it again with Tom!

Inside, Lucrecia was seething mad. *"This is not fixin' to happen! We will mess you up Tom. You have no idea what we are capable of when I am pi**** off, especially at a lazy man! We have had our limit, beyond our limit, of lazy men who are willing to watch as we kill ourselves as you refuse to lift a single finger. I will slow roast you over an open fire and smile while you scream in pain! You got that, Tom?"*

I tried to calm the demon voice within.

"Tom, I am surely grateful for our friends helping with the move. But I noticed that you did very little in the way of helping to haul the boxes or anything else for that matter. What was that all about?"

"I hurt Jamie. Look, I am older than you by fifteen years, and you expect me to move like I am your age. You are not even thirty yet, and I am forty-two. I get tired way faster than you do, and I am entirely out of shape. I weigh more than three hundred pounds, and you knew this about me when you chose to marry me. I don't see why it is such an issue with you now! Am I not good enough for you suddenly?"

"It's not that I am not appreciative of what you do for me and the kids. But I just get frustrated because it reminds me of Levi. He did nothing around the house, and I told you when I married you that I wanted a partner in this marriage. I am not interested in someone happy to point and bark orders. I had that for seven years, and I will not have it again. I will not live like that!"

This was our first real fight as a married couple, and it was the first of many, many more to come.

...

The Caboose Arrives

The kids and my mom arrived two weeks after Tom and I were married, and I had managed to get us settled into the new larger apartment.

We had decided to move Mom in with us to help me with the kids and the new baby. I secretly prayed that it would go better than when she lived with me and Levi. That was a bad situation, to say it nicely. I needed her help but did not look forward to her mouthiness. That drove me nuts!

On December first, I began feeling labor pains but I turned to Mom and said, "Let's 'go Christmas shopping.'"

She laughed and said, "Jamie, you're hurting. You're probably in labor. You can't be serious."

"I'm going … get dressed. You can come, or you can stay, but I'm going."

Within an hour, we were in Carson City, up to our eyeballs in Christmas shopping. I refused to allow her to push the shopping cart.

Finally, after a full day of shopping my contractions began to get real, I was at the check-out counter, bent over, writing the check out, and doing deep breathing exercises I had learned from *Lamaze* classes in Cincinnati. My Mother was pale with worry.

"Jamie, I figured this was going to happen. At least let me drive you to the hospital."

I knew that my Mom had no idea of how to get around the city, so I refused. This made her even more worried.

"I am fine. It just hurts a little. Call Tom and tell him I am in labor, and I am coming to get him right now."

When we reached Tom, he took one look at me and put the Explorer into overdrive with the emergency flashers on.

"Have you lost your mind, Jamie? I am not interested in delivering our baby *myself* in the Explorer!"

"Tom, this is my fourth birth. I have no intention of having this baby delivered anywhere but in the hospital. So, please just quit arguing with me and get me there!"

Within minutes we were being admitted into the hospital in downtown Carson City.

"How long have you been in labor?" asked the attending nurse.

"My labor began early this morning, about nine a.m. I was in Kmart, Christmas shopping when I began feeling the pressure a little over an hour ago... So here I am."

The nurse looked down at her watch. It was about five-thirty or so. I had been in labor since that morning. She didn't seem pleased about this.

"You went shopping!? Get this woman to a birthing room. This is her fourth child. She is probably close to ten centimeters already. Get her epidural ready!"

"I will not have an epidural and I do not want any pain medications at all!" I said loudly to the nursing staff as the nurse rolled me to my room.

The nurse asked Tom, "Is she serious?"

To which he replied, "Yes, she is very serious."

"Okay, well, let's get her into her room. Move it!"

As it turned out, my nurse was correct. It was absolutely time to deliver the baby. The doctor walked into the room and a few minutes later and with several hard pushes, Benjamin William David was born.

Tom was so excited he shed tears. He looked at my mom and said, "Oh my God, she is amazing. I have never seen anything so amazing in my entire life."

I was exhausted and emotional. I just wanted to hold my baby and sleep. I was so exhausted and so elated, all at the same time. I held my beautiful baby boy and fell promptly asleep.

It wasn't long after Benjamin made his entrance into the world that things went from bad to worse. None of us knew how bad things could get, but we were about to find out....

Chapter 16

The Investigation

A few months after Benjamin was born, I got a call one day from the Office of Child Protective Services (OCS).

"Hello, yes, this is Jamie, how can I help you? No, I had no idea that Jonah had a bruise on his leg. I just got home. Let me check into it, and I will get back to you. What's your number? Yes, I can call you back within thirty minutes. That won't be a problem at all."

What on earth is the OCS doing calling me? I worried. *And how did Jonah get a bruise so big his preschool teacher noticed it?* I was scared to death to look at Jonah's leg, but I knew I had to deal with it no matter how difficult it was going to be.

"Buddy, come see me for a minute. Let me look at your leg."

Unfortunately, there was indeed a bruise on his right side, just below his buttocks. My biggest concern was how did the bruise had been noticed by his school considering where it was located on his body?

I called the social worker back, and she set up an appointment so she could interview all of us—Tom, me, my mom, and the children. I was very nervous about this. I had never had to deal with the OCS before and was not at all excited about it. Around six that evening, the social worker knocked on the front door.

"Hi, Mrs. Herbert, I am Christine from the Office of Child Protective Services. I spoke to you earlier this afternoon. May I come in?"

"Yes, Christine, you may. My husband and Mom are in the living room. We were waiting for you. Would you like a glass of tea?"

"Tom, this is Christine, a social worker from the Office of Child Protective Services."

Tom made no comment, only nodded his head in acknowledgment.

"And this is my mom, Marie. She lives with us. The children are in their bedrooms playing. Would you like me to get them?"

"No, I want to speak with you three first. I am here because a report was made to OCS of a bruise on Jonah's upper leg/hip area. Have you seen the bruise?"

"Yes, ma'am we have."

"Can you explain where the bruise came from?"

Tom told her, "Ms. Christine, that bruise could have come from anywhere. It's a small bruise, and he could have fallen playing outside for all we know."

"So, none of you noticed the bruise before now?"

"No, ma'am, we hadn't noticed the bruise until it was pointed out to me by your office. I do have a concern. Considering where the bruise is on his body, how did the preschool teacher notice it?" I asked her matter-of-factly.

"She said that Jonah had to potty, and when she took him, she noticed it. She then reported it to her supervisor, who advised her to contact our office. They are mandatory reporters, you know."

Tom began to shift uncomfortably and angrily and interrupted, "I have things to do. Are we done here?"

"No sir, I'm afraid not. I still need to speak to the children. I will need to speak to them alone. Is there a place where I can do that?

"Certainly, the girls' bedroom is to the left, just beyond that half-wall in the den. Come, I'll introduce you."

"Tabby and Jonah, this is Ms. Christine, and she wants to talk to you both a little bit. Is that okay? She wants to be your friend, so y'all be nice and polite to her."

"Thanks, Mrs. Herbert. I will take it from here."

The Week from Hell

For an entire week, we were investigated by Child Protective Services, otherwise known as "CPS." The social worker questioned us, and I repeatedly questioned Tom. He continued to deny knowing anything. I was quickly becoming a basket case.

I cannot believe this crap! There is always some kind of drama I am having to deal with. Why in the he** are these people so concerned about a small bruise? I swear to God, I just want this sh** to go away! Just make it stop! And Tom's attitude is not helping. I could flush him down the commode and let him drown in his own filth right about now! If this lasts much longer, I am going to lose it on someone and go to the jailhouse! I know it! Just watch and see!'

I finally began to ask when it was all going to end.

"Mrs. Herbert, this is an open investigation," Ms. Christine informed me, "and it will not be closed until we can determine where that bruise came from. We have to be certain that the children are safe in your home. Their safety is our top priority. I'm sure you can appreciate that."

"Ms. Christine, I certainly can, and I echo that concern. I will cooperate with you as I have been, but I must tell you that I don't appreciate feeling like I have a gun pointed at my head each time I speak with you.

"You and your agency pose a threat to my family as far as I am concerned. I feel very violated that I was not called in first when the preschool teacher saw the bruise on Jonah's hip. And furthermore, I still don't see how she noticed the bruise in the first place. In my opinion, she was looking for something to pin on us.

"Tom mentioned to me how she looked at him when he would drop Jonah off at preschool. I'll bet it is the same employee who reported him. I think that she was intimidated by Tom's size and stern demeanor and when she found the bruise, in her mind, it was Tom's fault Jonah had a bruise on his hip.

"We are not a perfect family, but we love our children, Ms. Christine. My biggest fear now is who is going to protect *us* from *you*?"

I went on to describe the lady that Tom had his suspicions of from the preschool.

"Yes, ma'am that is the same lady, I'm sure. I appreciate your candor in this situation, and I will take your comments into consideration, but again this investigation will not close until we have an answer to where the bruise came from. We are not a threat unless we find reason to believe that there was ill intent."

One morning, a week later, my Mom was folding clothes at the dryer as I was loading the washer … and with no forewarning, she said "I hope Jonah didn't get that bruise from the spanking I gave him last week."

I quit loading the washing machine and faced her squarely:

"Mom, you *spanked* Jonah last week? With what?"

She left the room and came back in with a white leather belt. It must have been her belt because I had never seen it before.

"He was arguing with me and being disrespectful and he wouldn't stop so I spanked him."

She said it without an ounce of remorse as far as I could tell.

But that was about to change because she had no idea of how far I was willing to go to protect my children, even from her if need be.

"Mom, haven't I had this conversation with you? This is Carson City, Nevada. This is not Faubourg, Louisiana. Things are done differently here.

"I have asked you to come to Tom and me when the kids need to be disciplined. We don't spank the kids! We have other means of disciplining for this very reason.

"It causes problems! Sh** Mom. Now I have to call that social worker and tell her—after a week of denying any type of physical discipline—that you had spanked Jonah. *How could you? I should make you call her!*"

*WOW!!! This is just great! I swear I think I **hate** this woman sometimes. She has done nothing but cause problems as long as I have known her.*

After calming myself down, I called the social worker and handed my mom over to her. Tom was furious with me for telling about my mom's confession.

"You're going to pin this on your mother, Jamie? Are you out of your mind? I think we should get a lawyer and fight this."

"Tom, she admitted to spanking him and even showed me how she did it. Then she sent him to preschool like that and never said a word during this entire investigation. She deserves whatever she gets! I have told her repeatedly not to spank the kids. She never listens to me. I'll bet she does now."

The social worker picked up my Mom that same afternoon and took her to the police station to complete the investigation. By that night, she was back home—and clearly shaken. I offered her no support. She had it coming to her. She had me suffer through an entire week of questioning without so much as an apology to me or Tom. She could cry as far as I was concerned.

"They dropped the charges and gave me a warning. I am so sorry," she said, apologizing. "I should have listened to you. I was so scared they were going to take me from the kids that I couldn't tell you and I should have told you immediately. I never should have spanked him in the first place."

But the apology was a bit late for me. I was not able to let go of the fact that we had been investigated by the Office of Child Protective Services. It haunted me. I often had nightmares over the investigation. Mom, however, was able to go on and forget it as though it never happened. "Jamie, you have to get over it. It's in the past. Now let it go." I told her I was trying but it had just been so traumatizing for me.

On our date night one evening, Tom tried to encourage me: "You need to praise the Lord. He delivered us from the plan of the enemy." We were at Café Soleil in uptown Reno. I knew that I should have been enjoying the evening at our favorite restaurant. The food was excellent, and the atmosphere was very romantic with low lighting and soft background music.

"No, no I wholly agree with you. I am grateful to God for our victory, but I am still so angry with my mother. She watched me speak to OCS for a solid week and kept it to herself. I just don't see how she sleeps at night knowing what she did to me."

"Well, personally I just don't see how you could turn your own mother in to OCS. I still think we just should have hired a lawyer. By the way, those crab cakes look delicious. You should try them."

I picked up my fork, poked the steaming cake, and then set the fork down again. I had all but lost my appetite over the conversation.

"I believe in being honest. She did it, and she got what was coming to her. She spanked him knowing that I had asked her *repeatedly*, to let you or me take care of the disciplining of the kids. We could have gone to jail over her stupidity, Tom! Or, I could have lost custody of the kids."

Tom had the waitress put my food in a take-out box. "Thanks for the beautiful evening, Tom. I'm sorry I wasn't much as far as the company goes," I said as we walked out, arm in arm.

A night with you is always a pleasure. I just wish I could have distracted you better." He then leaned over and kissed me on the cheek before staring at the car.

"A night out with you is always a pleasure. I just wish I could have distracted you better."

He then leaned over and kissed me on my cheek before starting the vehicle to drive home.

The Last Straw

Lilly, my Mom's friend, and employer (a black woman who was middle-aged and hard-working), caught me alone at home one day. She had picked up Mom to go clean the house, and Mom had forgotten her glasses. So, Lilly left her to start the cleaning and came back to get her glasses. Before leaving, though, she asked me if we could talk for a minute. She told me something that helped me to see how rude and mean my mom really was.

"Jamie, for so long, I had such bad feelings towards you and Tom. All your mom ever does is dog you and your husband. She never says anything nice about either of you. She complains about everything you do for her, for the children, and about your husband, also.

"Then, one day, I thought about the situation, and it suddenly hit me. You and Tom have four young children, and yet she lives here rent-free. All you ask of her is to help with the upkeep of the house and watch the kids when you're busy. You tote her all over, and she never pays one cent for gas or anything, according to her own admission. She has it pretty good .... Girl; I don't see how you do it.... You are better than me."

I didn't say anything in reply, but after she left, my mind spun round and round with what she had told me. That was the last straw. I called our friends, Samantha and John, and within an hour, had rented a room for my mom in their large home, where they sometimes kept boarders.

I knew that the kids were going to miss her, but it was time for Tom and me to have a home to ourselves. We needed it. Having her live with us had caused so much turmoil. We needed peace of mind.

But still, I was so emotionally torn when she left. I loved her, but I couldn't stand her ugly ways anymore.

Jamie, you are evil, truly evil, I thought to myself as they drove off.

Chapter 17

These Crazies are God's People

As much as I wanted to feel relieved and go on with my life, I couldn't let go of the investigation and having to answer to OCS. I felt like a horrible parent who didn't care for her children or take the proper steps to protect them.

One night before bed, I called my sister, Kay, in tears. She had heard nothing of the investigation until I called her. I had been too embarrassed to tell anyone back home. She listened to me pour my heart out without uttering a word until I was done.

"Jamie, it's Mom who should be feeling badly about this, not you."

"I know that what you're saying is the truth, Kay, but I just can't shake this fear that it will happen again and I will lose custody of my children over it. I wake up in a cold sweat having nightmares over it. I feel like I am losing my mind, Kay … I am not coping and am constantly paranoid that something terrible is about to happen. I pray and find relief for maybe a few minutes to a few hours, and then bam! It hits me all over again."

"You are not losing your mind, Jamie. You're just a concerned mom who loves her children. Try to get some sleep, sis. You sound exhausted, and it's getting late. Love you, talk soon."

It helped to talk to Kay. After our conversation, I spoke to God about it too. "Dear God, please help me to get over the fear of losing custody of my children. Please strengthen my faith in you and give my heart peace."'

Night after night, I struggled. It came in waves. Some nights I didn't sleep at all, the anxiety keeping me awake all night, I worried that I might lose my children, and then I worried that I had done the right thing in the Lord's eyes by kicking my mother out.

Tom prayed for me—and with me, night after night, as well … encouraging me that the Lord had rescued us and our Heavenly Father was pleased with me.

"Jamie, you have to let it go. It is ruining you. You are losing weight and you look worn and exhausted most days. You have to put your trust in God that it is behind us."

"Tom, I was so scared that they were going to take my children and send them back to Levi and put Benji in foster care. Just the thought of that is more than I can bear."

It didn't help that Lucrecia was always there, berating me, making me second guess my feelings. *"You don't even like your kids some days, you liar! You would have gotten exactly what you deserved. What kind of mom sends her kid to daycare with a bruise on* *his leg? Then you want to cry 'waa-waa' when OCS comes. Tend to your business you irresponsible, lazy a**!"*

Tom continued trying to encourage me, "Jamie, how about a trip back home? You haven't seen your family in a while, and I know my dad would like to meet his grandson. Ben is old enough to travel now. What do you think? We could leave the two oldest with a sitter and take Benji and Gabby."

I felt like home was just what I needed—a change of scenery and time with my family. I was so thrilled to be going back home, even though most of our trip would be spent in Kaplan with Tom's dad. I would still have time to see my family.

I booked the tickets, and we took our trip in October, just after Jonah's fifth birthday. Benji was almost a year old, and Gabby would be three at the end of January. It was going to be a much-needed reprieve.

Louisiana, Here We Come

Tom's dad met us at the airport in Baton Rouge on Saturday, October 16, 1998, and drove us back to Kaplan. His dad, Tom Sr., was a very staunch man. He was quite proud to meet Benjamin, his new grandson, but he was not at all pleased with Tom. He and Tom exchanged words from the minute we got there.

He was unhappy with Tom for not coming to see him in Louisiana more than he did (which was understandable), and he had needed Tom's help. There was a strong feeling of disapproval in the home, and it attached itself to me. I needed to get out of there. My anxiety was worse there than it had been at home in Carson City and Lucrecia piped up again:

"The man hates you. He sees that you are not a good wife or mother.

He sees right through the games you play and the charming act you put on!"

By Tuesday afternoon, I had had my fill of Kaplan.

"Tom, I need to see my family. Your dad appears to be angry. I don't feel welcome here at all. I'm almost sorry we came."

"Jamie, he just misses my mother, and he misses, me, too. He would have been happier if I would have moved back here when she passed, but I have made my home in Carson City. He has never gotten over that. But I agree with you we need to see your family. Call Kay and see if we can all go and eat at the Catfish Place in Ville Platte this weekend. I know that they want to see Ben and Gabby and you too for that matter."

I called Kay right away.

"Hey Kay, we're in Kaplan. Tom wanted to know if you and Danny had plans this weekend. We would like to all go eat out if y'all are free."

"I would rather cook supper here for y'all. Jo wants to see y'all and so does Tante and Nonc. How does that sound?"

"That sounds great to me. We will be there Saturday morning and will spend the day. I look forward to it. Love you, Kay, and miss all of you."

We headed there early Saturday morning and spent the day. Danny had a roast on the grill and Kay had "dirty rice" on the stove and a potato salad in the fridge. It was going to be a great day. Jo had come in from New Orleans, where he had been living. The Cajun supper was great, and the company was even better. We all laughed and had a wonderful time. It was a welcomed change of pace. I needed the laughter terribly.

But after dinner, we had to head back to Kaplan. It saddened me to Be around Tom and his dad, who appeared to have a very strained relationship. It reminded me of my terrible relationship with my own dad and without warning, the anxiety returned.

As the trip went on, I was getting very little sleep and had completely lost my appetite. I was becoming delirious from sleep deprivation and Tom begged me to pull it together, But try as I might, it wasn't happening.

After two and a half days, Tom contacted Kay. "I need your help with your sister. She hasn't slept in over two days and isn't eating. She's almost delirious. Something is terribly wrong. She needs you."

"Jamie is Not Well"

I should have been humiliated by my appearance once Kay arrived. My hair was dirty and tangled and I hadn't changed my clothes in two days. I was not well.

Kay began to cry when she saw me and insisted, we go to Burger King to eat breakfast. I was an emotional mess, crying about how Daddy didn't even love me and how Tom's dad reminded me of all that. "Jamie, you need to calm down. You know that Daddy is just a hard man. He just has a hard time showing his affection. You can't let that get to you this way. Eat your breakfast. It will help you to feel better."

She looked away while she wiped tears off her face. Seeing me this way was hurting her deeply and I could see the concern in her eyes. Lucrecia noticed it too...*"Now you've done it. Look at you ... a blubbering mess in front of Kay. She probably thinks you're losing your sh** now with your homeless-looking self. Dirty hair, dirty clothes, weighing ninety pounds soakin' wet. You not haunt, girl?"*

That afternoon, back at Mr. Herbert's house, I found out Daddy was driving up to see me. I was so angry at Kay for telling him about my state of mind and felt so uncomfortable. This was no way to introduce Tom to my daddy. But, still, here he was, he and Mrs. D., and we had to deal with it.

This is just great. I complained to myself. *This is all I need right now. If I wasn't feeling nuts before, this ought to be the cherry that tops the cake!*

Daddy was not one to beat around the bush. "Kay called me. She is worried about you. What the he** is going on and why didn't you call me?"

"I am okay, Daddy. I was just upset. I am better now. There's no need to worry."

"You sure don't look okay. You're skinny as a twig and look like you haven't slept in days."

His direct approach was too much for me. Nothing had changed. He went on to have a conversation with Tom in French right in front of me. From the little I could understand he told Tom that he knew of a good attorney and could help him if I left him. He even went on to explain to him that he could sue me for reverse child support. I was mortified by what he was saying.

By the time Daddy left, I was completely undone. He had shown Tom exactly why he and I had such little relationship and had reaffirmed to me that he hated me and always had. The next day, I was almost completely disabled, barely able to speak, and paralyzed by anxiety.

My dad's behavior, along with everything else I had experienced over the prior months with CPS and my mother had pushed me over the edge. My father had humiliated me in front of Tom and his father. I wanted to vanish into thin air. I couldn't face another day of life on this earth. I had endured enough, more than enough!

Tom had also had about enough of it all, not knowing how to comfort me or help me, and assuming that I was *choosing* to fall apart in front of his father. "Dad, I am going to have to take my wife to the hospital. She has decided to have a nervous breakdown. I need to leave Benjamin and Gabby here with you while I take her."

We went directly to the ER in Kaplan where I was examined. I was able to give the doctor my name and could recall that I had four children, but as hard as I tried, I was not able to remember their names. I could barely speak from the anxiety and panic I was feeling, stuttering and stammering as I tried hard to answer his questions. Fear like I had never known before gripped my heart.

You are going insane, Jamie... and there's nothing you can do about that now. Nothing is going to stop it, no one is going to help you. You are going down... going down... down...

I was out of control, entirely, and at the mercy of the doctors in the ER. One of them picked up my arm and let it go— it dropped to my side as though I had become semi-catatonic. He ended the examination there and went to speak with Tom, where I overheard him say, "Your wife needs to be hospitalized in a psychiatric ward. She is on the verge of a psychotic break. When I examined her, she was semi-catatonic and couldn't even remember the names of her children. She needs help; help I am not qualified to give her."

That's when Tom called the airlines and cut our visit short— we were headed back to Carson City. "I need to get you back where the church family can pray for healing for you. You are not well."

"Okay" was the best I could muster as I looked around the room in disbelief, powerless to control any of it.

"Take Me to Jail"

Mr. Herbert drove us all back to the airport, but I still wasn't functioning in my right mind. At the airport, I was so out of it mentally, I left Tom to use the restroom and, on the way, back to him I noticed two security guards. I don't know what I was thinking, but I stopped them and said to them, "I need to be put in jail. I am not a good mother and have hurt my children. Y'all need to take me to jail."

Within minutes Tom and the kids were by my side and the airport security had surrounded him. He showed them our copy of the emergency discharge papers.

"My wife is not well. She needs to be hospitalized. We're going back to Carson City, and I will be putting her in the hospital there as soon as I can. As you can see, these children are in good hands and have not been harmed."

The guards looked over Gabby and Benjamin and let us go. "Good luck, Mister. We wish you and your wife the best."

Lucrecia was getting louder now. *"See Jamie, you're truly pathetic. What wife or mother does this? You wanted the police to arrest you and Tom …and what??? …* "Put Gabby and Ben where? … In foster care??? "You're so messed up!"

Tom was not happy with me on the flight home as it was his opinion that I had *decided* to have a nervous breakdown at his dad's house. He reminded me of this several times over the next six hours.

At one point during the flight, Gabby decided that she needed the restroom. I left my seat to take her to the bathroom at the back of the plane. Just as I put my hand on the doorknob, the back of the plane opened up and I watched in horror as the stewardess flew out. I was now hallucinating. Horrified, I ran back to my seat and put one of Benjamin's diapers on Gabby and told her to use the bathroom in the diaper. Then Benjamin woke up and began to cry uncontrollably as he had been teething and running a fever. Tom took the Benadryl out of the diaper bag and gave him a dose.

I looked at him and began to cry. **"Why are you trying to kill our baby?"**

"Jamie, I only gave him a single dose. He is only sleeping; he is not dead. Feel his heart if you are worried about him. You know he is not feeling well because he is teething. Why did you put Gabby in a diaper?"

"Don't worry about Gabby. She's fine. We just need to get home."

"I agree. We need to get you some prayer."

Shortly after our return from Louisiana, Tom called our pastor and a few friends to come and pray with me. I was no better after a week of being back home. I refused to leave the house, was barely eating, and had not left our bedroom. Our pastor, Pastor Tim, and a handful of friends and church staff came over to pray with me.

Ginny, a close friend of ours, came into the bedroom. "Jamie, how are you, honey?"

Her obligatory, "socially polite," conversation-starting question really hit me wrong, even making me angry, because I had not left my room in a week. Obviously, I was not well.

"Can we come in and pray with you, please?"
"Sure, I would love prayer."

Tom and Tim held my hands and Ginny sat on the bed with me. My mother came in and joined us, as well. "Father, we lift our sister, Jamie, up to you this evening. We ask that you give her the courage to leave her bedroom and we speak wellness and healing to her body and mind. … in Jesus' name."

Tom told me later that before he left, he was instructed by Pastor Tim, "If she is not up and around in the morning, I would take her to the hospital. She is not well and needs help."

The next day I did not get out of bed until noon.

By this time, I had huge dark circles around my eyes and had lost weight, now down to about eighty-eight pounds. I was wasting away and didn't care about anything. Even my children's needs were too much for me to deal with. I desperately needed help. Tom came home early that day. "You need to get up and get dressed. I am taking you to get help."

I got dressed but cried knowing I couldn't help myself any longer. I had tried to get well. I had asked for prayer. Nothing had helped. I was a mess. *What is wrong with you Jamie!?*

The Nut House

Tom drove me to Carson City General Hospital where I was admitted for a mental assessment and put on a seventy-two-hour hold for being a danger to myself.

I was so angry with Tom.

"You told me that it was just an assessment, and they wouldn't keep me. I don't want to stay here. **I want to go home**. I just want to be with my children. The people here are crazy. Take me *home*. … Please."

But that didn't happen. I was left there, all alone with all the crazies, to fend for myself—at least that's how it felt to me.

The Diagnosis

As I noted in Chapter One, I was diagnosed in the hospital with bipolar I disorder with psychosis. A person suffering from bipolar will experience a manic episode, during which they will have an extreme increase in energy and may feel on top of the world or uncomfortably irritable in mood; this mania may be followed by a major depressive episode. In some cases, the patient may also experience a break from reality or psychosis.

Mania in a person with bipolar disorder manifests as extremely upbeat, jumpy, or even wired behavior; grandiosity (an exaggerated sense of self-confidence); racing thoughts; extremely decreased need for sleep (may stay awake for days at a time and still have the energy to spare); and impulsive decision-making (such as expensive spending sprees, making foolish investments, taking dangerous risks, or spur-of-the-moment impulsive action). Psychotic behavior is defined as a break from reality where the person experiences auditory or visual hallucinations or delusional thinking.

My psychosis showed up plainly in the hospital when I expressed paranoia about my food, as I mentioned in Chapter 1. I honestly thought I was being poisoned by hospital staff and that they were trying to kill me.

Yes, I'm sure you will be quite happy to keep me locked up here so you can poison me to death, I thought wildly at one point when staff were trying to get me to eat. *Well, kill me if you must but I refuse to make it easy for any of you!*

I only started to come out of the psychosis and paranoia after taking the "cocktail" of medications I was given. I also began attending groups, sharing my childhood, poor decision-making, and the ordeal with OCS, which also helped.

And the vision of Jesus I had one night in the hospital certainly helped turn things around for me. In this divine revelation, I learned that the poor "crazies" in there with me were God's people downtrodden, helpless, needy," and I was one of them. "It is no mistake that you are here with them. You, too, need help," the Lord had told me.

Denial

While I accepted that I did, indeed, need help, I refused to believe that I truly suffered from "Bipolar I." As far as I was concerned at this time, I was depressed and anxious – "*downtrodden, helpless, needy,*" – and Jesus, the Great Healer, was going to cure me.

I spent Thanksgiving in the hospital and Tom and Benji were allowed to come and eat with me. I watched my son take his first steps at Carson City General. Now, how was that for therapy?

Nevertheless, I could not believe that I had actually had to eat turkey with my husband and son in a mental health rehabilitation facility—thinking about this fact did nothing to elevate my mood. I cried myself to sleep after they left.

After being in the hospital for thirteen days, I was discharged with the caveat that I would see my psychiatrist regularly, get involved in my personal therapy, and remain compliant by taking my medications.

This was going to be a tall order for me to fill because I believed with all my heart that I didn't need all that because Jesus was going to perform a miraculous healing for me. Who needed medication and therapy when Jesus could heal them?

Chapter 18

"I Am 'Healed' — in Jesus' Name!"

"Jamie, your medications *are not optional, they are essential* to your mental health and emotional stability," Tom furiously reminded me. "How many times do we need to have this conversation?"

Tom had discovered my medication bottles empty again after I had dumped their contents down the toilet. "I don't need them, Tom; I have already been healed," I told him. This was the third time he had caught me disposing of my medications over the last six months.

Desperate, Tom called our pastor. "Tim, she did it again. I don't think I can deal with this. I love her, but this is too much. Can you please come and talk with us?" Pastor Tim came over, though it was almost ten p.m. on a weeknight.

"Jamie, I know you believe Jesus heals," he said to me. "But you simply cannot proclaim yourself healed. You are not a medical doctor or a psychiatrist, or even a counselor. You need your medication. It is dangerous to de-medicate yourself. You must titrate off medication with medical monitoring. If you refuse to behave in a responsible manner where your mental or emotional health is concerned, you will be asked to step down from the ministry. I will not counsel you on this subject again."

Pastor Tim was a Godly man and one who was fair — but when he was serious about something, such as this matter, he could be pretty blunt.

I was livid with Tom for calling Tim — though I knew that I deserved it. It was so embarrassing to have a grown man chew me out like a child in my own home.

Are you happy now, Tom? Is that what you wanted was for him to give me an ultimatum? I will not be controlled, not by you and not by him."

"That's your choice, Jamie. But I will not continue to pick up the pieces you leave behind as you shatter yourself and our family. You are a mess when you're not medicated. You are emotionally unstable, a basket case, and have no patience with me or the kids. None of us deserve the ill-treatment you dish out. You scream and yell at me *for hours on end*, Jamie, over absolutely nothing. You're neglectful of the needs of the entire family. Hell, most days, I can't even get you out of bed and out of your pajamas. Is that really what you want to model for our children? When are you going to take the time to think about why you need your medication? Or are you the only one that matters?"

With that, Tom stomped off to our bedroom, leaving me to think about the weight of his words.

I realize that after this conversation, I should have known better than to de-medicate myself again. I wish I could say that I was suddenly responsible and had put it all behind me. I *wish* I could say that ... but I can't. Even though I would go a few months at least keeping my medication and not flushing it down the toilet, I wasn't necessarily taking it regularly. I was still listening to Lucrecia because, of course, she was always around whenever I had been miraculously "healed" and didn't need any of those pills!

"Jamie, you are so gullible. All I have to do is suggest to you that you are no longer in need of your meds, and you run to the toilet without even giving the consequences a second thought.

"Pa Ha Ha!

"Look at you, a crying unstable mess all over again. Tom is going to leave you!!!"

"I Will Behave"

Lucrecia had been having her way for several days, and I had not been sleeping. Tom had noticed I was becoming more agitated and finally had enough. He demanded that I swallow my medication in front of him before turning in for the night. He walked over with the Risperdal in his hand, which helped me sleep by shutting off the racing thoughts and demanded that I take it.

"Tom, please don't make me swallow that pill. I will behave, I promise."

I cried, curled up in the fetal position in our big king-size bed.

"That medicine is poisoning me, and I don't want to die."

My mind was telling me I was being poisoned, and I was convinced that the medication was killing me slowly.

"Jamie, this is your Risperdal. It is not poison. It is your night medication to help you sleep. It calms your mind and helps to prevent paranoia — which you are certainly exhibiting right now. The reason you think it is poison is simply the consequential paranoia you suffer when you don't medicate yourself. Please trust me. I would never hurt you. I am your husband. I love you."

But it was useless. I flat refused, out of fear, to swallow that pill. It was getting late, and Tom knew that the morning was going to come quickly, so again, he reached out to Tim for help. At almost midnight, he phoned him and explained how I was refusing to take that pill, and I was becoming psychotic. I heard the frustration in Tom's voice. Then he handed me the phone.

"Little Lady," Pastor Tim said, "if you don't swallow that pill, I will come to your home and force it down your throat just like I would a dog. I don't have time to argue with you. Swallow that pill."

Upon hearing these words from my pastor, I was even more fearful of my dire situation.

"Jesus, I trust you and I trust you to protect me from the poison that my husband is giving me tonight," I silently prayed and then took the pill from Tom's hand. Putting it in my mouth, I drank a big gulp of water and swallowed it down.

The next morning about ten, Pastor Tim checked in with me. "How are you this morning, woman of God? He asked in his usual positive voice.

"I am better; thanks for your patience with me. I didn't throw my pills away this time. I just didn't take them for a week. That pill makes me sleepy, and I hate that."

"I know, Jamie. I know you hate the side effects of your medications. I am curious, though, what made you finally decide to swallow the medicine? I thought I was going to have to shove it down your throat."

Tim and I had that kind of relationship. He was quite comfortable being direct with me, and I was the same with him. I trusted him. He was a Godly man, and I knew that his intentions were for the best.

"I said a silent prayer to God, Tim, and asked Him to protect me from the poison and then thought to myself, 'well when it's my time to go, I guess it's my time.' It was scary. I honestly believed Tom was trying to poison me … and you, too. As scared as I was, it was my faith in God's ability to save me from the poison that gave me the strength to swallow that pill."

The Definition of Insanity

I am ashamed to say, but it went on that way for years. Months would go by and I would take my medication and experience some semblance of sanity. I suppose if you call seeing visions of shooting your son in the head and then watching the bright blood drip from the small hole in his forehead sane and stable, then I was indeed sane and stable. Or, if you consider forgetting your daughter at daycare because you took a six-hour nap and woke up to the sound of the sitter knocking at your door with your child in hand … sound and stable … I was indeed sound and stable.

Honestly, I was not — by myself — fit for mothering my children most days. But thank God, I had Mom and Tom, who provided enough assistance and support so the children did not go without the necessities.

Then the "Lord" would "speak to me," and no sooner than I would hear His "word" declaring my healing (again), I would toss my medications and, again, begin my downward spiral.

Tim and our church family stayed the course with me and Tom. Each time we all suffered, but my children suffered the most. Each time I tossed my medication, they watched in horror as I turned into an emotional basket case, screaming at them, refusing to cook, neglecting housework, and my own self. They would watch from the doorway as Tom would plead with me to get dressed and brush my teeth to face the day, all to no avail until the Lord would get through to me again, and I would finally take my medication.

"Jamie, you are not well. You need to take your medication," my family and friends would tell me in chorus, sometimes four or five at a time. I'm equally ashamed to admit to this, but it took many of my loved ones to convince me when I was not well. Often it was the voice of the pastoral staff and their beautiful spirit-filled wives and other staff members whose voices God would use to bring me back from the pit of insanity.

"Jamie, your family needs you to be well," Treena, an Elder in our church and good friend, would tell me. "You have to fight the urge to de-medicate yourself. It's a part of your illness, Jamie. It's the medication that allows you to feel well and stable. You have to accept that."

Nevertheless, I believed strongly that, eventually, God would heal me from my illness, and I refused to consider that I needed a man-made medication to bring healing to my body.

Out of the Mouth of Babes

Two years after my diagnosis at Carson City General, my eight-year-old Tabatha asked me one day, "Mom, why do you yell at Poppa? It makes us all sad when y'all fight. And it is scary, too, because you get so loud."

"Tabby, I don't know why I yell at Poppa. Sometimes, I just get really mad, and it just comes out. I'm sorry. I'm sure I scared y'all. I love y'all, and I don't want to scare y'all. I will work on that."

"Okay, we love you and Poppa, too. Are you and Poppa going to get a divorce like you and Daddy did?"

"Tabby, you're sure full of questions today, aren't you?" I asked, looking into my child's eyes filled with fear and genuine concern … I looked away; it was too much.

"I love Poppa too and no, we're not getting a divorce. I am sick, and sometimes I don't take my medication and then I become frustrated and angry. I guess I take it out on Poppa and y'all too. I'm sorry for that, Tab."

"Yes, I forgive you, but if you're sick and your medicine helps you to feel better, why don't you take it, Momma?" Ahhh, out of the mouth of babes.

The question hit me like a ton of bricks, slamming right into my heart. I had no good answer for my intuitive daughter.

Yes, Jamie, if your medicine makes you better, why don't you take it? I cross-examined myself. *Because I am selfish and believe I know better than my doctors, Tab. That's why ... since you had to ask."*

"Come on, Tabby. Let's go and figure out supper for tonight. What do you feel like eating?"

I had straight-up wiggled out of the conversation that afternoon, but it haunted me for days, especially her last question, "... if you're sick and your medicine helps you to feel better, why don't you take it, Momma?"

With all the logical arguments I had used to convince myself I didn't need the medication, I couldn't utter one word in defense of my actions when faced with that question.

Yes, why, Jamie, don't you take your medicine if it makes you feel better? I thought over and over again.

Tom noticed that something was bothering me. "You're a million miles away, Jamie. What's going on with you?" He asked as I climbed into bed.

"No, I'm fine. Just tired I guess," I lied through my teeth.

I already knew his position. My medicine was "essential." I couldn't discuss it with him—I just couldn't bring myself to face the embarrassment of the illogical nature of my belief that only Christ could heal me.

At this point, I was wrestling to pin down this confused Jamie. She needed to realize that her family needed her to take her medicine. This Jamie needed to see her medication as essential. This Jamie *was* the problem. But this Jamie was in denial, not wanting to face the real demon within her. And frankly, it was time to knock off the crap.

But how?

How do you get a manic, psychotic brain to cooperate? That was the ten-million-dollar question of the day at the Herbert house and I just wasn't sure of the answer.

Do You Live in a Vacuum?

One night after a huge fight, I wanted to clear the air between Tom and me by trying to talk things out. I was not at all prepared for how that conversation would go, "Jamie, it has been two years since you were diagnosed. I have spent thousands of dollars on medical care for you, hiring babysitters, a housekeeper, and putting the kids in daycare so you can rest. Yet, I cannot see where you have made any significant progress.

"You still, to this day, see fit to sabotage your treatment by de-medicating yourself without speaking to your doctor first—as though you know better than your psychiatrist, who has a degree in this and has been practicing psychiatric medicine for over twenty-five years. I have had to beg you to take your medication as I watched you, in horror, lose your mental and emotional faculties, which you had worked so hard to gain in the first place." And he wasn't done.

"I have been accused of having an affair more than once, even with your own mother, for Christ's sake, Jamie. I have been screamed at for hours on end, called horrible names, and accused of trying to kill you, and you cannot see why I am upset about you wanting to help someone else other than yourself or your family. Do you live in a vacuum?"

By the time Tom was finished with his tirade, I was too upset to even respond to him. I put my head down and sobbed.

Despite how true his words were, I was in too much denial to see the pain I was causing him and the kids. All I was able to see was that I was trying the best I could and to Tom, it was not enough.

After about thirty minutes of self-absorbed tears, I was able to catch my breath and face him. But by then, he had gone to our bedroom and fallen asleep. This did not deter me. I was going to have my say. I flicked the light on and shook him until he woke up.

"No, Tom, *I do not live in a vacuum*. Most days, I fight the desire to stay in bed. I make myself eat because I have no appetite and the food has no taste to it. I am exhausted from being on five different types of psychotropic medications, and even a four-hour nap doesn't restore my energy. I just want to be well. I just wish God would heal me. I pray every single day for my healing, but for whatever reason, He sees fit to leave me this way. I don't get to live in your world, where there is no mental illness, and depression is a choice. It's not like I just decided one day to go crazy. I guess I don't understand your world any more than you understand mine. I have no idea where that leaves us. I don't even know if God can help us at this point."

That night I slept on the sofa, crying myself to sleep with tears of frustration, pain, and disbelief about the way my life was now.

I cried many tears that night, but honestly, that was because I hadn't discovered yet that I had the power to turn it all around. I was still too proud and self-deluded to accept the truth: that I was mentally ill!

The truth was I had been doing it all to myself. Jamie, the "psycho from hell," was in full control and doing a number on herself... her marriage ... on her family. But as she cried her self-deceived tears, this never occurred to her. Not ...At ...All ...!

Can We Talk?

After many days of deafening silence between us, Tom came to break the ice. He sat on the brown sofa right beside me and leaned forward, holding his head in his hands and choking back tears.

"Jamie, we have been ignoring one another for days now, I'm no happier about your mental illness than you are, but we need to get past this misunderstanding. Can we talk?"

"I don't know, Tom; let me see if I can manage to step outside of my vacuum to have a conversation with you!"

I was still pretty upset.

But we did manage to talk things out. We said our apologies and made amends to the best of our ability. I was very hurt, and so was Tom, but we were going to try to work it out.

To show how sorry he was, Tom lined up a date night. He told me about a movie the pastoral staff at our church had suggested called, *A Beautiful Mind,* starring Russell Crowe. Mom agreed to watch the kids for us, so we had a few hours of uninterrupted time to ourselves.

The movie turned out to be pivotal, a true game-changer for me and Tom. It was about a man suffering from schizophrenia, and through medical science, counseling, and the support of his wife and family, he learned to overcome his own personal struggle with mental illness.

I was moved to tears after watching this movie. It renewed my hope and Tom's too. I could use what I learned from the film to overcome my own mental health struggles. This had to be God saving me from utter destruction, I reasoned, because somewhere along the way, somewhere in my troubled childhood, somewhere in the hell that was life with Levi, somewhere... I had lost my way, and even worse, *I had lost myself.*

It was around this time that I finally stopped pretending I wasn't sick and started to face reality. It would take several more years before I got a true handle on my emotional health, but this marked the beginning of my long and arduous path toward true healing.

Right around the time Tom and I saw *A Beautiful* Mind, Pastor Tim introduced a new pastor to the staff. His name was Mickey Strickland. He was an ex-felon and had helped many mentally ill and afflicted individuals to overcome emotional illness through his keen understanding of how the mind works and how it affects behavior and choices. I was thrilled to have the opportunity to get to know him and his God-fearing wife, Carmine.

Mickey began to teach me the importance of taking my thoughts captive and ultimately learning to control my mind. To overcome any doubts about his sincerity in Christian leadership, I took his class "Breaking Through to Spiritual Maturity", and it was so powerful! Though I didn't fully appreciate it at the time, it would ultimately help me build the foundation I needed to become mentally and emotionally stable, which I will cover in greater detail…

Chapter 19

The Enemy is Among Us

One thing about the enemy he is a fierce and crafty opponent. It never occurred to me that the resistance Pastor Mickey had spoken of, that would come my way as I worked to bring stability and healing into my life may come within my own home, but it did! And it came from a very unexpected source: my husband.

After a day at school, I came back one afternoon to the sound of snapping and crying and walked into a horrible scene I will never forget.

"Tom, stop! That is enough! You're going to hurt him, and I will not stand for it!" I said as I witnessed him beating Jonah.

Tom had grabbed him by the arm and was lashing him with his leather belt.

"That boy needs to learn to behave himself and I am the one who is going to teach him," Tom retorted. "He is not going to disobey you or me while I am in this home."

Red-faced and with apparent determination, he was taking justified action, in his mind, for the way Jonah had disrespected me earlier in the day on the phone. Tom was quite intimidating, as he was no small man, standing six feet tall and every bit of three hundred and fifty pounds. The way he was handling Jonah was horrifying — like a rag doll. Tom had been a football player in college, so he was stout and strong despite his age. I must admit I was scared for Jonah and for me. But the fear did not stop me from protecting my son …

"Tom, you will stop now, or I will call Pastor Tim to come here, and I will tell him what you call discipline. Have you lost your mind? Don't you remember what we went through with Mom and OCS? Wasn't that enough for you? I ended up hospitalized over that!"

We had talked prior to this so he knew how I felt about excessive discipline. He and I had different points of view on what constituted discipline, and I knew this. Although it concerned me, I felt confident, up until this moment, that Tom respected my views enough to curtail his firm hand of discipline. I also knew Tom well enough to know that when he was in this mood, only Pastor Tim would get through to him.

"Of course, you will call Pastor Tim, 'The Great Savior.'" Well, Pastor Tim is not the head of this household. I will let your precious little Jonah alone, but when he becomes a problem, you can blame yourself for that."

He let Jonah go, and he ran to his room, red welts on his legs and choking back tears. He was being brave, but I knew that he was heartbroken. I knew it because I was heartbroken. The kids had told me that Tom would spank them. Mom had also told me. But until this day, I had not witnessed it for myself. I was completely horrified.

I screamed at him, angry and hurt.

"You will not lay another hand on any of the kids in that manner, do you hear me? If I find out that you laid into another one of our children like that, I will not only call Pastor Tim, but I will also call the law. It's abuse, Tom; it's not discipline, and you will NOT abuse my kids! You got that? Furthermore, I will not go to jail with you or for you!"

With that, I turned and walked upstairs to check on Jonah. He was sore and hurting but would heal in time, both emotionally and physically.

"Buddy, I don't agree with Poppa about the way he was spanking you. That was beyond what I call discipline. I'm sorry. But you need to be obedient. You were wrong to talk back to me. Poppa was trying to make a point that your behavior was wrong. Do you understand?"

Jonah was angry at me (and at Tom). I could tell. Head down; he nodded in agreement.

The Beginning of the End

The years that I had struggled with bipolar had for sure taken their toll on our marriage. Tom had tried to support me all through the times I wasn't taking my medication. He had worked hard to support our family and see to things at home when I couldn't function very well. I'm sure all this was very hard on him, and I noticed over time he became more and more impatient with me and the kids, and perhaps that's where some of the increasing feelings of rage that he turned on our children in the name of discipline had come from.

That awful scene was the beginning of the end for me and Tom. It only got worse from there in the Herbert home. As far as Tom was concerned, I had challenged his Godly authority, and he was not happy about it, not at all. I knew that was how he would take it, but I felt I had no choice in the matter. Someone had to defend the kids and it was going to be me!

I hated the distance between us, the constant smart a** comments from Tom, and his other taunting behaviors. He began to be very nasty to me and about me, saying things like, "Oh, the master has arrived at the Herbert home. Bow to the queen y'all." Our marital problems became noticeable to others, and we were approached by the Pastoral Staff with concern. Since we were in the leadership of our church, our family was not simply our business; it became the church's business as well. We had entered into a tacit agreement with church staff that our family issues were no longer our own private affair. Tom resented this but went along with it so he could remain a leadership position.

I admitted my concerns about our family to Pastor Tim:

"Yes, we're struggling. He is mad at me for 'challenging' his 'authority.' But I will not go through another investigation and lose custody of my children. He just doesn't understand or care that if you leave any marks or bruises, in the eyes of the law, that is abuse and not discipline. Not to mention, the kids do not require that type of discipline. They are not out of control. They are normal kids who need guidance … not abuse."

"I agree with you, Jamie, and I understand your feeling. Maybe I can help. I will try to talk to him. In the meantime, we will be praying for your family. The enemy is angry because of the progress you are making in your walk with the Lord and in your mental and emotional health, too. He is trying to destroy your family and, ultimately, your testimony. Prayer, Jamie, prayer is the answer."

"I agree. Pastor Mickey had told me just recently that there would be resistance, but I surely did not expect that it would come from my husband. I can truly say I did not see this coming at all. Please talk to him, Tim. He listens to you, and he respects your guidance and authority. I want my marriage to work, but I will leave if he continues to hurt the kids. I will not tolerate that from him or anyone else, for that matter. I turned my own mother into OCS to protect my kids. I will do the same with him if I am pushed, and he knows that."

Later that afternoon, after our church service, Tom approached me with questions about my conversation with Pastor Tim and was angry when I told him I had asked Tim for prayers and help. "Yeah, like I need the help of another man to save my marriage. That's a sad situation to be in," he replied in disgust.

Tom disliked the entire idea of having anyone in our business. He resented the help I craved from others. He had been raised an only child and was accustomed to dealing with things rather independently. He didn't want Pastor Tim's help, and that's when I realized my marriage was falling to pieces, and it felt as though there was nothing I could do to fix it. No matter how I chose to act, I felt damned either way I went.

Benji asked me one day as we were doing laundry.

"Mom, are you and my daddy going to get a divorce?"

"Benji, I don't think so. I love your daddy."

"Good because I don't want to live without you or him, and I don't want to have to move away. Daddy said that if y'all would get a divorce, you would take me back to Louisiana. I don't want to leave Carson City."

"Benji, we are working things out. Don't worry yourself about this. Pray and ask God to help us."

It was conversations much like this that kept me working on my marriage. The problem was Tom wasn't willing to put much into it anymore. He would not attend counseling and resented having to talk to Tim or anyone else in the Pastoral Staff about our problems. It hurt my heart deeply and caused me to often wonder if I had made another mistake in marrying him. *Where did I go wrong? Is this just another stupid mistake? Did I ignore all the red flags all over again?* Had I married a man who was just the same as Levi? And were both of these men replicas of my daddy? I had so much on my mind as I tried desperately to figure things out.

"Jesus, I need you more now than ever!" I prayed. "Please heal my marriage, my mind, my heart, and my family. We need you, Jesus. We need You desperately, and we need You now. I turn my family and my marriage over to you."

He Seeks Whom He May Devour

Even as our marriage suffered, thankfully, I became stronger in my ability to recognize my symptoms as a mentally ill wife and mother. I was so grateful to have support from the Pastoral Staff where my marriage and family were concerned. I knew that I was well-liked, as was Tom, as far as being Elders in the church. The staff recognized the spiritual gifts we were given to bless the body of Christ, both together and separately. This was a blessing and made us both feel encouraged.

This was very important considering how rocky our marriage had been over the last few years. We needed something positive and affirming. The staff supported us, and we knew it. But as time would prove, the support from the staff simply would not be enough glue to hold our home together.

Chapter 20

The Beginning of the End

No! ... Not our Pastor

One afternoon shortly after I had spoken with Pastor Tim about helping Tom and I work out our marital difficulties, I received a somewhat disturbing phone call from Pastor Mickey. He told me that something serious had happened in the church, and he asked that we hold a church leadership meeting at our home to address it. "Let me call Tom about holding a meeting here, and I will call you back," I told him. "Is everything okay, Pastor Mickey?"

"No, Jamie. Everything is not okay, but I am not at liberty to discuss it until we have everyone together. Call me back, okay?"

The meeting was set for Wednesday evening in our home. Time seemed never to pass, but finally, Wednesday arrived, and we were all gathered in our home. Pastor Mickey got right to the point of the meeting:

"Pastor Tim has fallen. We have removed him from his position as pastor/leader of the church, and he has been told not to contact anyone from the body at our church. We also took his cell phone."

"Oh my gosh! What happened?" I asked as I stumbled backward into a nearby kitchen chair. I knew that it was going to be bad, but this was not what I was expecting to hear!

"Jamie, it's a long story, but basically, Tim has fallen into sexual sin. And yes, Kristine is aware. They are currently separated. Tim left and is staying at a motel so Kristine and the kids can have their home."

"No! There must be a mistake. Tim and Kristine were so happily married. Did Tim admit to this?" I asked in disbelief and shock.

My mind and heart were screaming in unison: *'No, this is not right! There is a mistake! Someone got their wires crossed! Please say it isn't so!'*

Tom grabbed me up from my chair and held me to his chest while I sobbed uncontrollably. I couldn't believe this was happening to our beloved leader and Senior pastor. Surely this was the work of the enemy right in our midst! We, the intercessors, had failed him. The enemy had taken down a mighty man of God!

"Yes, Jamie and Tom, he did admit to it," said Pastor Ronnie. It happened last weekend with a young lady in the church. Tim openly admitted to having an affair with her."

Pastor Ronnie warned us all. "The enemy has taken down a mighty man. We need to lift him up and be in prayer for Kristine and the children. Now is not a time to be in judgment of Tim.

Now is a time to be in prayer and to remember that with the same measure we judge one another, that same measure will be used on to judge us. I warn each of you to be in prayer and be vigilant in seeking the Lord."

It's Only a Matter of Time ...

With Pastor Tim's fall, it was only a matter of time before our family followed suit. Tim had been the guiding force that kept us together and Tom and I both knew it. Without his leadership and guidance, I wasn't sure Tom and I could make it.

The morning after the meeting, I woke up feeling depressed and disheartened. *What is life going to be like without Pastor Tim in it?* I wondered. I just wasn't prepared for this change and without any warning! Despite my faith in my Lord, my heart trembled with apprehension.

I sensed that bad things were heading our way. So, I called up Pastor Mickey, who encouraged me.

"Be strong, Jamie. Keep your defenses up and be wary of the enemy. He is a fierce opponent and needs to be respected as such. Keep your eyes focused on the Lord, not the storm."

"It is a fierce battle indeed. Tom and I have been at one another's throats, and it has been awful without Tim to mediate between us. Tim had a way with Tom. Tom trusted him and respected his Godly authority. Now, he is angry, and there's no one to calm him when he erupts. It's been bad. We need prayer ourselves."

Mickey let me know that the leadership was behind us and would be praying for us. "Remember Jamie; we fight not against flesh and blood... Tom is not your enemy. Satan, himself, is your enemy."

As I talked with Pastor Mickey, I wept bitterly. My world was coming apart at the seams, so it appeared, how I needed God! I was a mess and as a mess I went to Him. Head bowed and heartbroken, I lifted my soul and pain to my God daily.

Day after day, I prayed for the church and its members, for the leadership team and their families, and for our family, our marriage, Tom, our kids, and myself.

Day after day, I waited for a sign that God was working on our behalf. I was exhausted and spiritually depleted as I lifted up the people I loved and fought the enemy, feeling as though I alone were fighting for our church, our families, and our marriages. Night after night, I lay beside Tom and prayed myself to sleep. And every morning, I would wake up praying.

This went on for months. I would let it all go at the foot of the cross of my Lord, and then I would take it all back again, worrying and doubting.

I won't lie; some days, I wondered if my prayers were falling on deaf ears. It felt like God was way off in some unreachable place. Tom gave no indication that he was seeking God. His attitude had turned from bad to worse, and he was growing colder daily. At the end of it all, I must admit my frailty. I am human, and I doubted God and feared my doubt would anger Him.

Walk by Faith, Not by Sight

Even though I was anxious and upset during this difficult time, it was also a time of growth for me. I was learning that my carnal mind had refused to see things from the spiritual perspective for such a long time. I knew I needed to focus on the fact that God Himself had allowed all the turmoil in my life to take place. God was not asleep when Tim fell with that young woman. God was awake, and He was aware. Yet, He allowed it. He wasn't asleep when I suffered as a child from my parents' cold, heartless, unkind ways. He was awake and aware, and He allowed it for a greater purpose. God wasn't asleep during my marriage with Levi when I made countless bad decisions, when I was deceived and mistreated by deceitful people... He was awake, and He was aware. And He especially wasn't asleep when I quietly descended into madness and lived among the crazies at Carson City General. He was more than awake and aware there... where he tenderly wrapped me in His loving arms and professed his love for the downtrodden souls in that horrible place, of whom I was one.

He allowed all of that in order that I might learn more fully how to come unto Him, to trust Him, to rely on Him, to believe in Him, and to eventually learn how to be truly healed by Him! But in the midst of all the turmoil with Tom at that time, I would not be able to see this. The realization of all that would come much later, as I will explain in upcoming chapters. What I was aware of this time was my absolute need of Him and that I needed to wait on the Lord for deliverance. That was all I could do at the time, just pray and wait.

Just leave it in God's hands, Jamie. Trust in Him, trust in the Lord, Jamie. This is how I encouraged myself after Tom and I would have another argument, and I would worry that we were at the end of our marriage.

When I prayed, it often left me exhausted and depleted, so I would take naps. My daily naps were one way in which I gave back to Jamie. I was not in the least bit apologetic for them. After one of our fights on the phone, Tom called back to apologize. I'm sorry, Jamie. I guess I just miss Tim, too, and I don't know how to cope with it. He was always there for me and listened to me without judging me. He understood me."

… This I could understand, and I was now listening to Tom with sincere empathy because my feelings were the same.

"Honestly though, Tom, we must learn how to control our tempers and try to get along because the kids pay for it. They worry when we fight. I worry too.

"You know I have Treena, Carmine, and Cathy to talk to regularly. But you have no one since Tim left.

"Can you please consider building a relationship with Pastor Ronnie or Pastor Mickey? I really think it would help you and us. Please pray about it."

Without having anyone to talk to, Tom stuffed his emotions, and then he would get angry and take it out on me and the kids. He needed someone on his side, someone to pray with him and listen to him. He needed a friend to walk through the fire with.

"I have been thinking about that same thing, Jamie. I will pray about it. You know I don't trust easily, and now it's even harder since Tim fell. But yes, I will pray about it. I need someone to talk to. I can see that."

I hung up and cried tears of relief over that conversation. It had been so long since I had heard any words of hope come out of Tom's mouth. I had to believe that God was at work. My marriage was at stake, and my mental health was not far behind.

I needed to somehow forgive Tom and learn to trust in him again. I had withdrawn since Tim had fallen, and Tom was getting the brunt of that.

I am not being fair to Tom, I reasoned. *I know in my heart that he is trying, and I have to remember that he is struggling too and has been since Tim left – Dear Jesus, please help me and help us.*

That evening when Tom returned home from work, we had supper together as a family and enjoyed one another's company. It was something we had been missing for quite some time. My heart felt so full as I absorbed the laughter and conversation at the supper table that evening. Surely God was working in our family. It was a beautiful thing to watch each child interact with the other with love and gentleness, just enjoying the peace of the moment. It was memories such as these that I lived for each day.

Chapter 21

Another Man Done and Gone

ut it didn't go the way I had prayed for the Herbert home. I decided to take the kids to eat out one night after a huge altercation between Tom and me. Again, we argued over the kids and our difference of opinion on how matters should be handled. Tom always felt that I was too lenient. My perspective was that we needed to show them love while still applying discipline. I tried hard to be fair and still firm.

Both Tom and I had come from the old school of thought where if you spared the rod, you spoiled the child. But I felt I had been shown mercy too many times by God to beat my kids half to death each time they made a mistake. They needed to be shown mercy, also.

I needed some space and hadn't been out with the kids alone in ages. It seemed like a good idea at the time. So, we went to our favorite eatery in Carson City and sat together in our favorite booth at Chilis.

It felt like the makings of a great evening, and I desperately needed that at this time. I was beginning to feel relaxed as we ate our appetizers and casually asked the kids, "So, how are things going for my little rug rats?"

I often referred to them by this term of endearment and various others, such as, my little demonios (de mon iooos).

"Well, kinda good, really; at least we no longer have to suck Poppa's toes," Tabatha replied. "I don't know what happened, but I am just glad."

Instinctively I fought back the urge to faint right there at the table.

"Can you please repeat what you just said for me, Tabatha? I don't think I heard you right."

"Yes, I said that Poppa hasn't been asking us to suck his toes anymore since you have been home more. And we haven't been spanked in a while either."

I slowly set my fork down while trying hard to hide from the kids that I was dying inside, and my world was spinning like a top. I experienced sudden tunnel vision –suddenly, there was no one else in the room but me and my kids. The chatter from the other customers was instantly miles away.

"So, you haven't been spanked in a while either? Well, uhm, when was the last time? I guess y'all have been good then, huh?"

It was taking all the strength I could muster, but I was trying to normalize the conversation. I knew that if I sounded angry or shocked, they would clam up. I learned this while working with juvenile delinquents at Sage Winds as an addiction counselor in training. When they were divulging their secrets, it was imperative to listen intently and keep it normal.

"It's been a while, Mom, like about a month, I guess," said Jonah. "And I am sure glad because it hurt. He would make us scream into our pillows so you wouldn't hear us crying."

Jonah seldom had a problem with telling things just the way they were. He was a lot like his Mom, direct, matter-of-fact, and honest in his details, normally without exaggeration.

"So … Poppa would make y'all scream into a pillow, Buddy?"

I was beyond furious at this point and having a really hard time with remaining calm.

"Is there anything else that Poppa did while I was not around that y'all would like to tell me … since he is at home? We can have a pick-on-Poppa night."

I was trying to make it a little lighthearted, but I was feeling more and more sick to my stomach, and more was shared with me.

"Mom, he did a lot of stuff," said Jonah, "but he said if we ever told anyone, he would beat us silly and divorce you. So, we never told anybody."

I was dead inside by this time, but I pressed forward. I needed to hear as much of this as they were willing to tell me. Something kept me feeling as though I needed to question them more, although it was making me nauseous to hear it.

"Tell me more about having to suck Poppa's toes. Did you really have to do this, and did you *all* have to do this or just you, Tab?"

I really could not believe my ears. *What the he** was this fat a**hole thinking having my kids suck his toes? Sweet Jesus, this man is going to die tonight,* I was thinking as I listened to my kids go on to explain the numerous times he, indeed, had them suck his toes.

"He was usually at a friend's house when it happened." I still remember the taste of the fuzz from his socks," she went on, "in my mouth. We would try not to, but he would say that it was that or get a spanking, and it hurt when he would spank us."

Tab expanded on Gabby's response. She was the oldest, and I could see she was uncomfortable talking about the toe-sucking. I was beyond horrified. *Who does this??? Who in God's precious name makes a kid suck their toes???*

The sickening information continued during that conversation and I knew right then and there that my marriage was over. He had gone waaaayyyyy too far, and I had to protect my children. It was time to get into mama bear mode, exit my marriage, and defend my children.

I hardly touched my supper, I mostly just moved the food around on the plate, but as hard as the evening had been, I was so thankful that I had decided to take the kids out to eat. Obviously, this was a meal that was long overdue.

It made perfect sense now why Tom always insisted that we eat together as a family when I would mention taking the kids out to eat alone. I never fought the issue because I respected his position that mealtime should be shared by all of us. He certainly knew how to work me. I had fallen for his ploy to keep me from speaking to the children alone, and they had suffered for it long enough …

Tom was a clever man, probably one of the most intelligent people I had ever met. He often used his wits to demean people without their even being aware that he was putting them down. He enjoyed being a step above those who could not compete with his intelligence. It gave him a sense of superiority, though he wholeheartedly denied that when I called him on it.

But for all his intelligence, he was no match for the wits of God. The Word says that what is done in darkness shall be brought to the light. This night was God's Word in action.

We left the restaurant late and drove up the winding hill to our very large, four-thousand-square-foot home on Comstock Drive, overlooking the city and the university. I didn't even notice the glimmering lights or the star-filled sky that night. I was too distracted by the events of the evening to notice anything but my need to get my kids in a safe space, away from the monster I had married — the monster I still loved.

I instructed the kids, in hushed tones, barely above a whisper as we sat parked outside the house: "Go upstairs quietly, pack a bag, and then get back into the car. Do not talk to Poppa. We're going to go to a hotel tonight. It will be a sleepover. I will call Poppa and tell him once we get there."

This was easy enough to do since the staircase leading to the kid's bedrooms was in the front of the house and the master bedroom was in the back. If they were quiet, they could enter through the front door, get their things, and leave without him ever knowing.

He Needs to Die

When in the car alone, I called an ex-police officer friend I had worked with at a previous job as a rehabilitation skills counselor at Nevada Rehabilitation Center.

"James, I know it's really late, and I apologize, but I need you to listen to what my kids just told me."

I told James in detail what I had heard and ended with, "I can see the guns in my head. I know exactly where they are, and they are loaded."

My voice was stable, and I felt a sense of peace come over me as I spoke to James. I was suddenly very calm and focused. It was a weird feeling and not a familiar one.

"Jamie, listen carefully to me. I know how upset you must be. I would be too, but you cannot raise your four children from inside a jail cell. Come to my house. You and the kids can spend the night here with me and Rachelle. You need to be with friends right now. Get a pen and write my address down."

With great reluctance (and with the kids and their bags now in the car), I backed out of the driveway and headed to James and Rachelle's home. Once there, James took my Colt 45 from me and put it in his safe. I had a concealed carry permit and plenty of training in handling a weapon, and I always carried one with me when I left home alone or with the kids. He also took my keys for safekeeping. I am grateful to him for his foresight. I might have gone back there that night if I'd had the opportunity. I had never in my life felt such rage, and it the desire to hurt Tom was almost overwhelming.

I said to James and Rachelle from the safety of their sofa — and from the bottom of my heart,

"Thank you for listenin' to me. I think I might have made a huge mistake if I hadn't called you. I will never be able to thank you enough for being my friends and letting me and the kids sleep here for the night."

I knew that the Lord had led me to call James. But my blood was still boiling as I dozed off to sleep. Still, I was safe, and even more importantly, so were the kids, and that was something I hadn't felt in a very long time. I had become so accustomed to living in such a dysfunctional state that I never realized I was actually living in fear. None of us did until we slept away from Tom that night.

The next morning, after calling into work to take the day off, I called Child Protective Services and with a heavy, grieved heart, did my duty and reported my husband for suspicion of child abuse.

It was taken very seriously, especially once I told them that I was a mandatory reporter and worked with troubled kids in the area as a rehabilitation skills counselor for the Nevada Rehabilitation Center.

Rachelle and I dropped the kids off at school and went from there directly to the police station, where I made a report.

Reporting Tom was the right thing to do for my children, but it was the end of my marriage and life, as he, the kids, and I had all known it.

Chapter 22

Score—For the Enemy

fter I reported Tom, I felt sick to my stomach, emotionally depleted, and utterly defeated. In my mind, the enemy had won. He had destroyed my family, and I had allowed it. Some prayer warrior I was! I felt as though I needed to apologize for my inability to protect my very own children.

The man I had married had harmed them and had done so right under my nose. I never even suspected it during that time. As much as we fought—and fight we did—I had trusted him not to bring harm to my kids. I knew we had our differences, but it never occurred to me that he would hurt the kids to spite me.

But now I believe that is exactly what took place. It is said that hindsight is 20/20. I don't know about that, but I do feel that it is easier to see a situation for what it really is once you've been able to put some distance between yourself and the events that trouble you. I see now that Tom was angry about having to share me with my children and having to support me through a mental illness and not able to take his anger out on me because he knew I would leave him, and because of that, he took it out on my children.

Which explains why only Benji never had to suck his toes. It was no coincidence that it that the toe-sucking only took place when Ben was at a friend's house. He wanted to demoralize my children and make them pay for my wrong doings in our marriage. He was fed up with having a bipolar wife. It was his way of making them feel subservient to him. Truly, he was a sick man. But God was going to take care of Tom.

I needed to focus on getting help for my hurting family.

I should have sought out help for me, too—I needed it badly. I think, looking back, that I went back to many of my bipolar behaviors after this event.

Lucrecia came back with a vengeance. I was angry—angry at myself; angry at Tom; angry at the world, and, without a doubt, angry at God. I began self-loathing and got right back on the path to self-destruction. That evening at Chili's the demise of Jamie began all over again, a huge part of me died that night—. The naïve and trusting part of me believed that there was good in everyone, but it was laid to rest that night.

I had lost Pastor Tim and I had turned Tom over to authorities to be investigated. Bad things were happening to us, but I still believed we were good people. My heart was ground meat, and my foundation was being violently shaken.

All together and all at once, I felt

- that there was no escaping this massive storm,
- that I didn't have the faith to keep my eyes on Jesus rather than on the storm,
- that God, my Father, had abandoned me in my time of need,
- that He had closed His eyes or looked the other way when Tom was hurting my kids,
- that He had allowed it to happen,
- that He could have stopped it,
- but that He didn't.

When I thought of this, it caused me to hurt so deeply that I had chest pains and shortness of breath.

Where was my loving God when Tom was spanking my children and they were having to scream into a pillow?

Where was God when my children were having to suck his toes?

Where were you, God?

"Damn you Tom Herbert. Damn you straight to hell!"
Lucrecia screamed inside my head.

I had no idea where to begin to forgive myself, Tom, or God. I was too consumed in hurt and hatred to worry about forgiving, but I did worry about my ability to survive all of it.

Jamie, we will make it through this! I think I can. I think I can. I think I can, I would tell myself over and over.

This became my mantra as I fought hard to keep from descending into bipolar hell. I was certain it could get no worse…

And then, it did!!!

"Jamie You are Not Worthy"

One Sunday afternoon after Pastor Ronnie had preached, he stopped at my home to check in on me and the kids.

He had also come to set some things straight. So when we were away from the children, he said to me, "I think it is best if my son, Jayden, doesn't come to your house anymore. Jonah is welcomed to go to ours, but until things die down with the investigation with Tom, I think it is best if the kids visit each other at my home."

The blows just kept a-coming. It was not fixing to let up. The enemy was having a field-day at our expense—mine and my kids'.

WOW! How the mighty had fallen. My home, where numerous church events had been held, had become unfit for the pastor's son to visit. What's worse is that Ronnie was right, if I am to be completely honest.

I had taken to drinking and frequenting bars and casinos with a female co-worker and friend of mine. She was a great support to me in my desperate time of need, dragging me out of the bar and driving me home when I was too far gone to do it myself. There were many a night we cried together, she and I, over the condition of my life and the pain I was living—me and my kids.

She was an employee at the new job I had taken in Carson City as a rehab counselor (ironically enough) and had heard my story. She had been in a similar situation, and we quickly became close friends. Her support meant the world to me and the kids.

I needed her support, as life as we had known it with our many friends and church family had been suddenly thrust into the abyss in a matter of a few weeks. Tom was being investigated by both CPS and the Carson City police department. I had to evict him from our home so the kids and I could return to it—I could no longer afford hotel fees. I also put a temporary restraining order on him, and this made him very angry. Naturally, I felt threatened by him. On top of that, the pastoral staff had somehow decided that because Tom attended church, they needed to distance themselves from us also.

Pastor Ronnie had chosen to minister to Tom. I had heard through the grapevine that Pastor Smith had shared his opinion that I was being "misled" by my children who were being "deceptive and cruel."

Apparently, no one had chosen to minister to me or my children.

In effect, my kids and I were abandoned by our church family.

It was all too much for my hurting, grieving soul. And since I was so angry with God, I turned to alcohol and carousing for comfort. I must admit that during that time, I was not stable, and my children suffered for it. It was a dark time in my life, and I was troubled. Troubled is a kind word for my state of mind. I was a devastated mess. I was grateful for my four children. They provided me with the motivation to wake up and face another day. They kept me from going off the deep end and never returning. They thought they needed me, but in reality, I needed them just as much as they needed me or more. My sanity was being seriously tested and my spiritual life had all but ceased to exist.

I knew that God was still on my side, but I had chosen to live as though there was no God. I was convinced that He had failed me and my kids and that I didn't need Him. I think that I even hated Him at times — if I am to be totally honest. I blamed God for the condition of my life and my marriage. I had trusted Him, and this is where my trust had taken me! I didn't need that kind of Higher Power! Thanks, but no thanks, God!

If the emotional toll wasn't heavy enough, there was the financial aspect of it all. To pay the mortgage and feed my children, I had to sell many personal items that I hated to part with and wouldn't have under different circumstances. Still, I was standing in quicksand and quickly losing the ground beneath me. I needed help desperately.

I was working two jobs at this point to make ends meet. By day I was a rehab counselor, and by night, a hostess in the Atlantis Casino.

Tom had furnished the great majority of our income, but since we were separated and he had been evicted, he offered no assistance to pay the mortgage. I began to realize that I couldn't afford Carson City if I was going to be a single mother of four growing teenage children. But I had no means of returning home to Louisiana, either. I was in a dilemma and had few support options I could turn to.

About six months after the separation, the children and I had to leave our beautiful family home on the hill overlooking the city, traipsing here and there, hither and yon. I got no monetary support from Tom for Benjamin and only sporadic financial contributions from Levi, and that was only when I called him to beg and demand his help. Although I didn't see it then, I am fully aware today that it was solely by God's good and bountiful graces that I was able to keep my children fed, clothed, and together during this hard, devastating trial.

More than once, God sent one of his followers to buy us food and bring it to us. What a God I serve! In the midst of my anger and ugly outright rebellion towards Him, He summoned people to bring food to me and my children.

My friend Elaina is just one example of the Lord's kindness. As we were preparing to eat a few biscuits one night, the doorbell rang, and Elaina was standing there. "Come with me to my car and help unload the groceries; I have food for you. I heard the Lord's voice and He said to buy you food. So here I am."

She walked over to the fridge, opened it up and saw that it was bare, and said, "Yes, He was right." Then turning to me, she continued, "The Lord told me that your cupboards were empty. Well, they're not anymore."

Our food was often provided by the local food pantry. Once, a kind stranger purchased our entire cart of groceries from his own pocketbook because I was broke and crying at the register. We made it—but by the skin of my teeth. I did get food stamps, praise God, but they did not last the month. And it was slim pickings when they ran out, and I had to purchase our food.

My children were wonderful and brave. At the young ages of fourteen and thirteen, Tabby and Jonah found jobs shaking advertisement signs for $10 an hour after school and during the summer. They also used their hard-earned money to purchase their school supplies and clothes, and even provide food for the entire family during the lean times.

Jamie is Self-Destructing

With the trouble and the drinking came more trouble in the form of men. I picked up a boyfriend or two during this time and got picked up more times than I care to admit. If I am to be entirely honest, I had lost just about all sense of moral scrupulosity, \or even *concern* for right from wrong.

Everything became blurry morally when I thought about Tom supposedly loving me, attending church with me, and hurting my children while leading the worship team.

Screw being a good girl... what good has that done me.

I rationalized that the wrong I was doing was justified by the wrong my family and I had endured. I, like so many, was in a state of denial and needed my Savior to rescue me from myself and my hideous path of self-destruction.

Worst of all, since my health insurance had expired and I had no way of paying the premiums, I was without my mental health medications. I was vacillating daily between mania and depression, often experiencing both at the same time. I recall many week-long periods of sleeping for hours on end, followed by severe spells of insomnia. I almost completely lost the ability to parent my four children during this time.

Praise God that they were good kids and did not stray from the truth they had been taught. Otherwise, I would have had quite a challenge on my hands as a single mom of four, angry with the world and running from her Maker. I was angry on so many different levels that even my few remaining friends and family members couldn't believe the person I was becoming.

"Jamie, hi, it's me, Cathy," one of my best friends from Carson City inquired. "I have been so worried about you. I wish I wouldn't have moved so far away. How are you dealing with everything, honey? I miss you so much!"

Cathy and I had raised our children together and also cried together over the loss of our church and Tim. She and her new husband had decided to move to Indiana on a leap of faith to start a fresh new life. I surely missed her. She was one of my biggest fans. Maybe the distance helped with that. Lying through my teeth to her, I told her I was doing okay and still trying to trust in God. "The case with Tom was dropped by the D.A. for insufficient evidence. I was pissed, but there is nothing I can do. I wished he would have gone to jail," I admitted to her. "I'm doing okay," I hated lying to her but was too ashamed to admit to how far I truly had fallen.

I Can't Do This Again

With the passage of time, despite the deep rage I felt toward Tom, I considered trying to forgive him. It took some work to come to that conclusion, but my desire to be right before God led me to it. I had broken up with my then-boyfriend, Guy, and thought that perhaps forgiving Tom meant also taking him back. Boy, was I wrong!

While Tom and I discussed giving our marriage a second chance for a short time, it went nowhere. God quickly revealed that there was too big a gap in the way we each saw discipline in child-rearing, and I was not willing to live in fear for my kids. It was simply not an option.

Once I realized that God wasn't in it and that it was over between Tom and me, it was easy to see I needed to return home ... to the South, to my roots, and to my family.

"Goodbye, Tom. I won't be staying here in Carson City. It's too hard for me as a single mom here. We're moving back to Louisiana. We aren't going to live in fear of your temper — that behavior was completely unacceptable."

Yeah, and you can consider yourself lucky I don't find a baseball bat and beat the sh** out of your fat a** for scaring my kids like you did.

Tom didn't think I was being fair but, he could see my mind was made up. "Just please let me see Ben before y'all leave. I would like to have some time with my son."

Tom then reminded me of a retirement policy that had accumulated about $25,000 in value. I cashed it in and split it with him. This was my ticket home and a miracle from God.

I called Kay to tell her I was moving back to Ville Platte. I hadn't spoken to her in quite some time and there was plenty of catchin' up to do.

"Get the gumbo pot ready. We gone be makin' a trip back home. And this time … it's for good. I will be sending the three kids first to stay with Levi, until I can get everything set up here for me and Ben to follow."

Kay was speechless … but finally said, "Well, it's about time. Just let me know when I need to put the gumbo goin'. I'm ready me."

Chapter 23

Sweet Home Louisiana

Ever feel like you're trying to fight your way out of a paper bag and the bag is winning? I have had days when I couldn't have won even if the paper bag was soakin' wet.

The recurring theme in my life has always been trying to fight my way out of something that I have got myself into in the first place. And once again, as I prepared to move home to Louisiana, I got myself into a fix again (surprise, surprise).

I wanted to reach my arm through the phone line and strangle his pathetic, freckled-face self. But I knew he was just being vindictive.

Another Mistake

Knock. Knock, I heard one afternoon at my door. "Jamie, I heard you're leaving Carson City?" My ex-boyfriend, Guy, was at the door.

"Yes, you heard right. I can't afford this city. It's too expensive here. I need to put myself in a place where at least I will have a fighting chance.

"What are you doing here, Guy?"

"Jamie, I have had a while to think about our breakup. I love you and I want another chance. I miss you. I miss the kids. I am willin' ta change. You were right; I was selfish and lazy. But I can change that."

"Don't do it, Jamie. He is a part of your past, Lucrecia warned me. *Leave him there, idiot!"*

"Can you think about it?"

(Me, thinking for a minute.)

"NO! Jamie, I told y..."

"Well, I could certainly use a second driver. Are you up for a long trip, and we can see how it goes from there?" I told him.

"Crap, here we go — you've done it again!"

And just like that, I had gotten myself into another mess.

Guy helped packed up my house, and I gave a lot of stuff away. We just took the furniture and the essentials. Everything else got left behind. The truck was packed like a sardine can. It was the beginning of a new life for me and my kids, and would you believe it? *Mardi Gras* weekend?

After many days on the road and an unexpected detour through New Mexico and Texas, we finally made it to Louisiana. We pulled in about three Saturday morning, completely road-worn and ready for bed. Kay was up with a pot of gumbo waiting just as she had promised. *"Mais la!* (Look at that!) It sure took you long enough," she said. "I tried to call about a million times and was getting worried. I thought you had decided to go back to Carson City. I can see ya'll are tired. I'll heat the gumbo, and then ya'll eat and get to bed. We can visit in the mornin'."

And did I sleep??? I think we all died a little that night.

It was so good to be on Louisiana soil again. I made myself a promise that night that I would never leave my home again unless God Himself told me differently.

The next few days were filled with family and catching up. My kids came to visit from Levi's. I got to see Tante, Aunt T, Parin Ray, (my Godfather and Aunt T's husband), and many of my cousins I hadn't seen in years.

Nonc had passed while I was living in Carson City and I went to visit his gravesite and bid him my farewell. I sure missed Nonc and our good times. It was sad thinking about my children never knowing him. The rest of the weekend passed way too quickly, and I had to take the kids back to Levi's.

Reality Sinks In

Reality sunk in quickly as I realized I needed a job. The trip had taken quite a bit, and my money was running low. Praise God for food stamps. That kept Ben, Guy, and me in sandwiches and milk and within a week, we had a place to stay at Kay and Danny's camp. It was far from a palace, but it had a roof, running water, and two beds.

All I wanted to do was get a job so I could move into a better place and have all my kids back under my roof.

I began applying everywhere I could think of and then some. My Bachelor of Arts (BA) in Criminal Justice had to mean something to someone, right? I tried the local jail, the sheriff's office, probation, and parole, and even checked with the lawyer's office in Ville Platte... Nothing.

One thing I had forgotten was how hard it was to find a decent job in Ville Platte, Louisiana. But I was praying and believing God would provide.

And provide He did.

The first miracle came from Tom, of all places. He had gotten on disability and called to tell me to file for a check for Benji. "You should get half of what I receive monthly," he said. This was truly an answer to prayer, and I immediately hit my knees and thanked my God for His provision. But God's supply didn't stop there...

The second miracle came when the office of medical records in Ville Platte called about a job as a support coordinator. "We are impressed with your resume. Can you come in for an interview?" I was elated when two weeks later they offered me the job.

Again, God was answering my prayers. Many of them. I laid my head against the sofa and let the tears of relief streaming down the sides of my face. "Oh my God, thank you, Lord Jesus, for your provision."

The job involved scheduling and supervising the physical and mental health care needs of disabled individuals. I got some quick training, received my caseload on a Friday morning, and by Monday, was traveling down dirt roads with no signs to name them.

The directions to the homes of the individuals I would be visiting had given me were crazy but typical for small town Louisiana: "Turn down the road with the white fence that is half broke, go about 200 yards den make a quick lef', and we live back yonder way, behind the blue and gray house with the large front porch, watch out for them dogs, yeah, call when you get dere and we'll go meet you at the car".

I chuckled to myself as I listened to the sorely missed language of my Cajun folk. I knew that it wouldn't be long before I fell right in with them and the Louisiana slang. I loved being home!

It was a blessing having a job and money, but things at the place Guy and I shared were anything but blessed. Even though Guy had been working for my dad and had proved himself to be a good worker, he was finding more reasons to drink and fight which did not make me happy. He resented the long hours I had to put in at work and the late nights. I had to remind Guy how I had moved home to start a new life and find relief, not to be unhappy with his complaining. *Hadn't Lucrecia tried to warn me?*

One Sunday night, after getting home late from helping Tante, Guy shoved me to the ground, and my cell phone went flying. I had no way of calling out. Ben had gone on to sleep over at a friend's house that night, so I was alone and at the mercy of this fool who had been drinking and probably shooting up, too. He demanded to know where I had been. He caught me by the hair and swung me around hard, slamming me into the bedroom wall, leaving a huge hole in the sheetrock. He then shoved my nose into my face with his fist before I could even begin to fight back. Once I got my footing, we tussled, and I began to bleed profusely from my nose. That scared Guy, and he backed off. "Jamie, I am so sorry. I was mad. I just lost it," he pled.

But it was too late for apologies. It was over for Guy and me. The next day I filed charges against him. This situation caused some serious issues between Daddy and me. Guy went to my dad's house to drop off my Jeep the next day, which he had been using. He began running his mouth about how I should have been home with him instead of out helping Tante. My Daddy, being the great father, he had always been to me, took Guy's side and the next day told me he was ashamed of me and no longer wanted a relationship - that I was an embarrassment to him. That was March of 2008. We haven't spoken two words to each other since that day.

I never spoke to Guy again, either, but I did see him hitchhiking his way out of the state after he was released from jail about four months later. I guess you could say that the third miracle God gave me was getting Guy out of my life, something I wouldn't have needed Him for if I had not gotten involved with him again in the first place.

God continued to bless me, even in the midst of all that, and the fourth miracle he performed was being able to fight for and obtain custody of my kids from Levi. We were able to all be back together, living under the same roof.

It was a beautiful blessing to have all my kids with me again. It was also a bit scary financially, but I had to believe that God was capable of supplying our needs the same way He had done in Carson City. Between my job, child support, and God's grace, I had faith we would survive.

Chapter 24

Is it Another Train?

ou never know when life is going to throw you a curve ball. I had become accustomed to ducking a punch or tucking and rolling from being thrown from a moving vehicle so to speak, but this one I must admit I did not see coming. Just when life was becoming calmer and I was becoming more stable, the light at the end of the tunnel was yet another locomotive heading my way...

Months later, on my job, I was driving to one of my client's homes when Tom called, yelling at me about some nonsense. I was in my red Mustang convertible at the time. The next thing I remember, I was waking up in an ambulance with my head throbbing pretty badly and feeling engulfed in fear.

"I'm hurting. Am I going to be okay?"

"Miss, you've been in a pretty bad accident. We're taking you to the hospital. You just rest now."

When I woke up a few hours later, Kay and all of my kids were gathered around my hospital bed in the Intensive Care Unit

(ICU) of Lafayette General Hospital, looking very concerned. I was in a lot of pain and was hooked up to an IV pain relief drip.

Reading my mind, made plainly visible by the confused look on my face, Kay explained to me, "You were arguing with Tom on your cell phone, apparently, and pulled out in front of a truck that was doing about sixty-five. You are lucky to be alive, Jamie. You almost made it, but he T-boned you on the driver's side The man is okay, but your car didn't make it. It was banged up pretty bad. You hit your head pretty good but they're going to release you in a few days." On your driver's door window, and you have a good-sized knot on the side of your head."

"I believe that, my head is killing me," I said feeling the lump on my skull.

It was hard to talk because the pain was so intense. As I spoke, my head throbbed. I laid back onto my pillow and my world began to spin a bit. I was weak and hurting, but thankful to be alive.

"Y'all can go home. I'll be okay here until they release me. I know you have to work, and the kids all have school."

"Jamie, they have told me that it will be weeks to months before you are able to drive again—or return to work," Kay said. "You're going to need some help with the kids. I called Mom. She is ready to move back down. I have purchased a plane ticket for her. She will be home this weekend and will stay with the kids until you're well."

I passed out then and slept for hours.

I have no other recollections of my hospital stay. Even what I am relaying to you now, in large part, is coming from stories told to me.

I was released a few days later, but still with aches and pains. I had broken my collarbone on the left side and was pretty bruised up. But the worst was the headache. I was also suffering from a tremendous amount of anxiety. I vaguely recall any of the events after that for weeks. I was released on painkillers, and they caused me to sleep, a lot.

Within a month or so I was ready to return to my job, or so I thought. However, after two weeks on the job, it was painfully obvious I had returned to work too soon. I couldn't remember anything and my ability to focus and concentrate had gone out the window. I had to call the office every two hours or so for the address, directions, or my schedule. Tonie, the CEO of the company, called me into her office at the end of week two and told me she didn't think I was ready to be back at work. She put me on leave and told me to go back to the doctor.

"You know, before the accident, you had thirty clients and were handling the caseload with no problems. That was the most difficult caseload we had, and you were doing it without assistance. Now, your caseload is half of what it was and you're struggling to keep up. We're not upset. We just feel it is best for you to heal more."

I left Tonie's office both relieved and discouraged. I had to agree with her— I was struggling. But I needed to work. I needed the money. And I also needed the distraction. But I resolved myself that the Lord knew best, and I would have to be patient a little longer with my healing.

My anxiety became more pronounced as the weeks went on, which was dreadful. I was struggling with driving and having flashbacks of the accident when I did try to drive. My family was concerned and so was I. I had never had a concussion before and was afraid that the short-term memory loss would be permanent.

I was a walking nightmare. I had to put sticky notes everywhere to remind me of everything because if a minute passed, I forgot where I was going or what I was doing.

On top of all this, I hadn't been taking my medications for bipolar disorder in years because I had no money for the insurance premium. I had managed to keep things "under control" all that time but was dealing every day with a serious mental illness without medications. Now the pain medications I was taking were affecting my thinking and I started into a downward spiral. Although I had returned to work for a couple of weeks, which did help, I still wasn't able to get my footing under me.

Before I knew it, I was spending hours locked in my bedroom, refusing to come out unless it was absolutely necessary. No one knew this (which I kept *very* private), but there were days I prayed for God to take me home. I felt so lost and useless. Mom was helpful with the kids, but only a miracle from God could save me from the abject depression and insurmountable anxiety I felt at this point.

At one point, my body felt as though it weighed a thousand pounds. Try as I might, I had no motivation and no energy to do anything. Even getting out of bed and dressing for the day was too much. I wanted desperately to be well and feel happiness again. If I could have willed myself into good mental health, I certainly would have. I was sick and tired of being sick and tired. I cried until I wasn't able to cry anymore.

The tears had dried up. It was very frustrating as I had four teenage kids who needed their Mom. And I knew this. Aside from that, I needed to work but had no motivation to fight the depression on my own. My accident had really set me back and I was suffering the consequences of it daily. My family was suffering with me and yet I was powerless to do anything about it.

"Jamie, nothing, not even God can help you. If you wouldn't have been arguing with Tom, like an idiot, you would be fine right now,"

Lucrecia screamed at me. *"Look at you, hair a mess, don't even want to get dressed for the day, and your kids need you. When are you going to get your sh** together? Your kids deserve better, and you know it."*

I lay there feeling guilty but was powerless to do anything about my declining emotional health. What most people fail to understand about mental illness, especially clinical depression, is that it's not a matter of being weak-willed or lazy. It goes far beyond that. It is a despair that is deeper than the deepest abyss, that settles into your heart and mind and takes you captive. The disabling nature of any kind of mental disorder is hard for anyone not suffering from it to understand. Before I was diagnosed, I judged people such as myself in ignorance:

Now I lay in bed, hoping and praying that God would give me the strength to face the day. Mental illness is real. After all, who in their right mind would *choose* to feel this way?

It's not a choice.

It's not an excuse.

It's not a weakness.

It's an illness and it's very real.

I kept praying and asking, no begging, God for His help. It was all I knew to do because I was losing it. I was sinking into a clinical depression. I recognized the signs. I had been there before...in Carson City... the hospital with the downtrodden.

I can't go back to that state of mind again... I can't... I can't....

Let's Jitterbug!

One Saturday in late September, six months after the accident, I was feeling pretty good and had been having a few decent days in which I had left my bedroom, cleaned the trailer, and even cooked supper. Kay called and said, "Let's go out tonight. I have a bunch of friends who are looking for a ladies' night out. I think you could use a good time."

Miraculously enough I managed to stir up the courage and went with Kay and her friends. It turned out to be the best decision of my life.

That night in September of 2008 I finally met the true love of my life!

We were at the Jungle nightclub, and he walked up slowly to the truck, lagging a little behind his drunken friends who were already crowded around the truck. He was smiling as he looked at me. I was sitting in the back seat and leaned out the back window, three sheets to the wind, and slurred, "Heeeyyy, I knowww youuuuu. We went to school together."

"No ma'am, you have me mistaken for someone else. We are about ten years apart. But my name's Brent."

Brent and I danced all night, and he was a perfect gentleman. He had long, darkly tanned, muscular arms and was a great dancer. His hair was light brown, wavy, and long and he wore it in a ponytail. He had a blue jean cut-off shirt on and looked good in his Wranglers, I must say.

He taught me to Jitterbug that night and I bellowed a Loretta Lynn song in his ear—perfectly out of tune in my excited state, and filled to overflowing with shots, JD and Coke, and way too many beers. I had not had so much fun in a very long time. It was a night I needed. He and I danced until I was sweating and exhausted.

About three a.m. the bar closed, and we all went our separate ways. But on the way home, we stopped to help a couple of women who had too much to drink and had taken the ditch. But we were unable to pull them out.

Lo and behold a big, white F-150 pulled over and out stepped Brent. Our eyes locked, and I walked over to him and put my arm around his waist and walked him over to the two ladies who needed assistance. It felt so natural, as though we belonged arm in arm.

I was shocked to have seen him again—but also relieved. He had driven away from the bar without us exchanging full names or numbers, but this time I didn't let him get away. I took his silver flip phone and entered my phone number in it. With a drunken smile, I replied, "Here you go, Brent."

That night would change my life forever... I just didn't know it at the time.

Ring. Ring. "Hello, Darlin'"

"Hi, Jamie? You know who this is?"

"Uhm, no, I can't say I do."

"It's Brent, the guy from the bar the other night. You put your number in my phone."

I immediately went crimson. "I did do that, didn't I?"

"Yes, you did, and I am glad."

Hmmm, you poor foolish man. You have no idea who you are about to tangle yourself with. You need to listen to me and RUN! RUN, boy, RUN – and don't look back.

He didn't run. But unlike those who had preceded him it was the beginning of a truly genuine friendship and a beautiful romance. He was every bit the gentleman he had shown himself to be at the bar, on the dance floor, even with the ladies in the ditch!

Like me, he was separated from his spouse of twenty-four years. He was living in Grand Prairie, and his wife was in Texas with their nineteen-year-old daughter and their grandbaby ("All-ll-ll my ex-es live in..." oh, never mind you, know the rest).

We talked that night and the night after and the night after that into the wee hours of those beautiful mornings. I enjoyed our conversations and laughed often. He was therapy to my soul. I didn't feel in the least bit threatened by him, and he was a great listener, as well.

He was always there when I needed him and never went more than a few hours without checking in on me and the kids — in a good way that left me feeling warm and cared about. He made me feel special, and I hadn't felt like that in a very long time. He respected my boundaries and treated my kids with the same respect he did me. This meant the world to me. He had a bit of a crazy streak in him, but he knew when to put on the brakes.

Brent also believed in God and had a relationship with Him. We talked about God often, and he prayed for me and with me. He proved to me over and again that he was someone I could count on, someone who filled a need in my life. "You must be one crazy man for getting involved with a woman with four teenage kids," I said to him one day. "You now, we are all a bit square. I don't party much. I hope we don't bore you to death."

"I like kids. and I like *your* kids," he gently replied. "They're good kids. You're a good mom to them, and we get along well."

Brent was just what I had been needing in my life. He was very patient with me and supported my decisions.

"Thank you for being so supportive. You never make me feel like I am beneath you. I like that."

"Jamie, you will never be beneath me. I am looking for a partner, not a servant. I want someone to live this life with. You are an answer to my prayers, Jamie."

And he was an answer to mine— a blessing and a Godsend— both to me and to the kids. We all needed each other. He had experienced a rough life with his previous two marriages, and so had I. We had a lot in common. It was good to be with someone who could relate.

I was far, far from perfect with this mental illness I have," I confessed to Jerry one day. "I was simply being human, but aside from that, I have come to realize that God was not first in my previous marriages, and that's a lot of the reason they didn't work. He will need to be first in my next one if it is going to work."

He admitted to me that he had been no saint with his ex-wives.

"In my younger days, I was hell on wheels, and no woman was going to tame me. I did what I wanted to do and didn't much care if they didn't like it. But with you, it's different. I don't feel as though you try to control me, and I appreciate that. You make me feel like a man."

Brent was very supportive and understanding of my illness. He never made me feel crazy and had great compassion for me.

He encouraged me to return to work, yet he understood my anxiety about driving.

He was a painting contractor and had his own business. He taught me to paint, and I went to work with him to pass the time and deal with my anxiety. I tried to work day job but it was too much for me and I quit due to anxiety over driving.

Eventually I was unable to drive at all. So, I was very grateful to join Brent on his painting jobs from time to time, which got me out of the house and prevented me from ruminating on how I was going to pay the bills without being able to work. God knew what I needed. Brent was amazing. He helped financially with what I was not able to make to keep me and my kids fed and the bills paid.

It's All a Shitstorm from Here

Despite things going well for me in my personal life and my finances becoming more stable (with Brent's help), my mental health symptoms began to spiral downwards. I was sinking deeper and deeper into depression and anxiety.

Once again I refused to leave my bedroom. Fear would grip my chest when I thought about leaving and often, I had panic attacks. I was becoming a prisoner in my own home. I sent Brent, Mom, or the kids to do the grocery shopping,

"I'm so sorry. I know that you didn't sign up for this," I told Brent in tears one day. "I don't know what to do. It scares me to death to leave my bedroom, but I know that I can't live my life this way. I feel so bad for you and the kids. Y'all don't deserve any of this."

"Jamie, I am here, and I am not going anywhere. We will get through this," he comforted me. It will get better, you'll see."

By this time, Brent was living with me and the kids and was basically providing the income. I stayed home, locked in my bedroom, while he went to work and the kids went to school. Mom tried to coax me out, but she seldom managed to succeed.

Each day, Brent, Kay, my mom, and the kids became more and more concerned over my condition. Brent drove the kids to school and/or picked them up. The kids helped to pick up the house and keep the chores done. Mom cooked.

Me? I was losing weight and my mental health was quickly deteriorating.

I was hanging on by a thread at best. Jo and his wife came to check on me occasionally and although I appreciated the thought, it did no good. I was more embarrassed to be seen in my state than it was helpful.

I looked like a hag—to put it nicely. My hair was constantly greasy and dirty, and I shoved it into a baseball cap to hide how awful it was. I might have showered once a week—if Brent begged me enough out of pure concern. This went on for almost a year, until Easter Sunday. It was an uncharacteristically good day for me. We went to Kay's and the kids all enjoyed themselves. But I told Brent and Kay I needed to be evaluated for another inpatient stay.

- I was having suicidal thoughts again and could barely make decisions for myself.
- Brent or my kids had to reassure me that I had chosen the right outfit for the day.
- I would cry over having to get dressed.
- It was too stressful to think about fixing my hair and facing the day.
- I just wanted to sleep in the darkness of my cave and be left alone as much as possible.

All these things were disturbing to me, but what happened a few days later really cemented for everyone the fact that I desperately needed professional help.

Look at the Little Doggie!

I was on a job with Brent in a neighborhood in Houma. I sat out in the truck and played on my phone while he painted inside. When he came out to check on me about mid-morning, I said, "Baby do you see the little doggie chasin' the butterflies in that field? It's such a pretty spotted doggie. Do you see it?"

Brent's face became flushed, and he said to me in a concerned voice, "Darlin' come and sit in the house with the air conditioner on. You need to get out of the sun a minute."

"What's wrong?" I asked him. "Did I make you mad or something?"

Brent stared at me a moment and then reluctantly replied,

"Jamie, there's no grass or field. We're in a neighborhood and there's cement everywhere. There's no field and no dog and there are no butterflies. Please try to rest a minute. I think you are hallucinating."

I was pretty scared then, as I saw the concern on Brent's face growing. I had seen this look before. It was in Tom's eyes when he begged me to take my medications and I accused him of trying to poison me.

"Okay, I will try to take a nap. I'm sorry. I didn't mean to worry you."

Lucrecia's voice was coming through loud and clear, "*You stupid b****! I told you not to lose your sh** with Brent. He is good to you. He is good to us. How you gone go and act this stupid with such a good man? Get it together, Jamie! Or you will lose him for good!*"

Noooo.... not again, I found myself pleading after the incident with Brent and the imaginary doggie and butterfly. I was risking a psychotic break with reality but didn't want to face the horror of having to be admitted to a psych ward at the hospital. *I don't want to be with the crazies again.*

But like it or not, Lucrecia's angry voice was getting louder and louder, and I was getting further and further away from sanity. I was terrified of this possibility as much as I was having to go back to the hospital.

"*Don't mess this one up Jamie!. Get your sh** together before Brent sees how crazy we really are. He's a good guy and he is good to you and the kids, but he won't stay if you show our full crazy to him.*"

I couldn't argue with Lucrecia. I knew she would end up calling all the shots if I let things go any further, so finally, the Monday after Easter in 2009, I asked Brent to drive me to the hospital in Lafayette. After an extensive evaluation, the doctor recommended that I be admitted for an inpatient stay. I agreed, but then cried my heart out at the thought of having to be hospitalized again.

I had promised myself that once I was released from Carson City General, I would never go back. Yet here I was, starting the whole nightmare all over again.

But this time, I knew what I needed to do.

I took my medications without having to be told and no one had to convince me I wasn't being poisoned by the staff. I participated in group therapy willingly and wholeheartedly. I listened as they shared their stories and empathized with their struggles. I took pages and pages of notes in my composition book which Brent had brought to me.

I invited Kay, Mom, and Brent to participate in family day in the unit. This gave them an opportunity to speak to my therapists and ask questions about my diagnosis. It was a bittersweet day as I was so grateful to have their support but sad that I needed it in the first place.

Having a diagnosis of bipolar I disorder with psychosis is no joke. I was beginning to see why Dr. Rizzle had been quite bleak with me about my prognosis eleven years prior at Carson City General.

But there was one thing that Dr. Rizzle and all the textbooks didn't know about, and that is the power of God, Yes medical professionals, medication, and good therapy play an important role in the *managing* of mental illness, but there is only one source to which we can go to tap into the power of actual healing—the God of Heaven and Earth, the Lord and Savior, Jesus Christ.

Along with Him, the kids and Brent were my saving grace through all of it.

In the hospital, I was making progress and felt myself gaining strength with each passing day. I was so grateful for my progress that I praised God for my decision to go inpatient. Whether I liked it or not, my medications were my saving grace, and I could feel the difference within a few days of taking them again.

I felt the presence of my God there, stronger each day. He was healing me. I could feel it and I had never been so grateful for my mental health as the day they released me. I knew that never again would I take my mental health for granted.

Looking back, I can see that there were many times I had danced on the edge of insanity. It was only by the grace and love of my Father that I had not lost my way entirely!

Chapter 25

Jamie is NOT Well!

By August of 2010, almost eighteen months after being hospitalized, I had almost completely recovered. Every day I was gaining more and more strength, stability, and mental clarity. I felt great most days and praised the Lord that I was no longer a prisoner in my own body.

My relationship with Brent was wonderful and we got along fabulously. I had never been happier in my whole life as I was at that time. I smiled a lot, from the inside. And it was a real smile, not the fake one I started pasting on as a child to cover the pain of the emotional turmoil at home, or the one I used to hide the pain of being married to Levi and Tom. This smile expressed genuine happiness — it was a heartfelt smile that reflected my true peace of mind.

= I was rocking my life! I had a routine that include daily self-care. I fixed my hair and put on make-up, whether staying home or leaving the house. I kept a clean house (well for the most part considering that there were eleven of us living under the same roof!), and I kept the bills paid. The kids were growing well and doing fine in school.

I felt such happiness about actually being present, living, no longer feeling like I was a spectator, watching myself go through the motions of living, without really living.

But most importantly, Lucrecia was gone.

For the first time in many years, her sadistic personality no longer lived within me. I said goodbye to her, and good riddance, accepting myself for who I am and choosing to be happy just the way I am, foibles and all.

When I think of all that it took to get me to a place of actual healing, I am sincerely humbled. Looking back on my life, I was so selfish in my recovery. First of all, I was too proud to admit that I, Jamie, in all her glory, could actually have a debilitating mental illness—a challenge that I couldn't master by myself.

Even with all the trauma I experienced as a child in a toxic home, and everything I suffered as an adult, I had always been good at overcoming, or at least I thought I was. In reality, I wasn't really overcoming anything... I was actually a slave to mental illness and hid behind Lucrecia's ferocity to appear able to handle it all. I had been beaten for years! I was a slave to bipolar disorder. It was my master. But no more. I am learning to master it so it no longer controls me.

Brent was so happy to see me happy, back in school in pursuit of a master's degree, and driving myself there no less.

"Baby, I am so proud of you. You have been doing so well," he said to me one day. "You are taking good care of yourself and the kids. It makes my heart so full to see you smiling and enjoying life. I love you and I want to marry you and spend the rest of my life with you as my wife."

"Awwwe, I love you too darlin'," I replied. "Each day I thank God for you and the kids. Without your support I wouldn't have made it."

On August 1 of 2011, Brent and I tied the knot. It was truly the happiest day of my life.

Thirteen years later I am still having the "happiest days of my life." That's because I live in gratitude for all my Heavenly Father and His Son have done for me.

I no longer feel like the shadow of the person I was. I feel like a better, stronger version of the person I am meant to be. I can make decisions on my own. I can drive without fear that I will kill myself or someone else. I don't have flashbacks or panic attacks anymore. I can talk to a total stranger without fear or anxiety. I can spend time with my kids and enjoy their company without feeling overwhelming guilt wash over me. I can pray and not wonder if God is actually hearing my prayers. I enjoy spending time alone with Jamie as much as I enjoy spending time with my family.

I don't despise myself anymore, and I no longer have Lucrecia in my life to torment me. I put her to rest. I no longer feel as though I am an outcast in my family of origin.

I must admit, my life is rather boring and mundane now, but this mundane life is exactly what I have been searching for all of my far-from-mundane life. I no longer go to bed worrying about what tomorrow is going to bring. I no longer wake up crying because I am terrified to brave another day on earth All my life I have only wanted to find "normal," to feel like others... to be like others. I know now that we all fight our own personal battles involving all kinds of problems. No one is "normal!" But I must admit I don't miss all the drama that my life with mental illness brought me. Today, just living in the moment and enjoying every mundane minute of every mundane hour is sheer heaven for me.

And though my life is rather "normal" now, what does make me unique is that I have chosen to face my demons head on. I may have suffered in denial for longer than was necessary, but I no longer pretend that I beat these devils with anything other than clear, objective thinking, and through the help of trusted professionals, and of course my God.

Today, I point the finger at my demons and say "You will not keep me down. I have risen from my ashes, like a Phoenix. I have overcome!!" Jesus worked miracles through prayer and ordinary means. when I finally let Him.

So today, I am shouting from the rooftops, "I am well! Praise God; I am well!" Do I still have my bad days? Of course, I do, but they no longer keep me captive in fear.

I no longer fall to pieces and become immobilized when I am faced with a difficult situation. I have learned to face each day on its own terms and not borrow trouble from tomorrow. I am not trying to say that I am perfect at it. I won't find perfection until I meet Jesus face-to-face. But I am learning to walk upright on my own two feet and with little to no assistance.

Yes, I still take my medications. So, yes, I recognize that I have not yet been fully healed. But I have also accepted this as God's way of keeping me humble and appreciative of what others can offer me.

Like the day that Mrs. Joy told me how amazed she was by the person I was becoming and how much her offer of gracious support meant to me. "Jamie, you have overcome so many obstacles in your life and yet you still smile and find it in your heart to be kind to strangers," she had said to me before her passing. I hugged her tightly and thanked her for her kind words; it was such a blessing to hear them. I never thought in my lifetime I would have people speaking praises for overcoming the challenges. It seemed that I was going to live my entire life burdened and slumped over. But that was not God's plan for me.

And it is not His plan for you either!

Don't put this book down just yet! Read it to the last page and absorb the message God has in mind for you. Take what you understand He wants to give to you from this book. It is my belief that if you are reading this, it has not been by accident. God has a plan for your life just as He has a plan for mine. I am joyfully in the process of working out that plan.

Are you? Could you be?? Why not???

Chapter 26

My Journey to God

re you comfortable? … Here, let me fluff your pillow. How about a glass of tea or fresh-squeezed lemonade? Or even better, how about a cup of Community Roast coffee (with two scoops of sugar or the sweetener of your preference and just a dab of cream or your favorite flavored creamer)? Whatever your choice may be, I am inviting you to join me as we embark on the last (but best) part of my journey — the revelation of God's plan for healing me, which may ultimately help heal you.

I'll be very honest with you (like I haven't been thus far, huh?), this is hard for me to do. So please forgive me if I stumble around for just the right words to express what is going on in my heart right now for you. I feel I have laid myself and my life open before you and you know way more about me than you may have ever wanted to. But I haven't yet shared my heart with you in its entirety — the part of my heart that has to do with you and your future.

This memoir has not been simply a means for airing all my dirty laundry. No, I have written the book because I felt God called me to do so... for you, and struggled with that fact for about three years before ever putting a single word on the page. I lamented the arduous job to which I had been commissioned.

However, I never could have dreamed it would be as difficult as it has been. With each word I have prayed that the message I have been called to give you has been well received, even among the shocking details of my life,, my dear reader. I have done all this for you because believe me, I know what you are going through!

My hope is that as you've waded through the muck and the mire of my life, you've been asking yourself:

Does any of this speak to me?

Does any of this resonate with my soul?

Can I relate to what this author has written at all?

And I truly hope that you've found yourself answering:

"Yes It Does!"

"It speaks to me ... here."

"It resonates with me here ... and here."

"Oh, boy! Can I ever relate to this ... right here!"

Because if you have resonated with the book, then my job as an author has been fruitful and I can rest knowing that my desire to reach you through the painful process of baring my soul has been worth the sacrifice.

I must confess that I am no longer the Jamie Brown Guidry Herbert "Freis" Goudeau who struck that first keyat the beginning of writing this book. I am a stronger and much more compassionate version of that woman than I was when I began its writing over three years ago. There's an ache in my heart that wasn't there prior to beginning this book.

And that ache is for you, my friend. I long to see my words act as a means to help transform your life. I sincerely desire that like me you can experience God's healing power to overcome whatever it might be that you suffer with, and that as you do. I hope you will share your testimony with me and others about God's healing and transformation in your own life. And now that we are almost finished walking this path together, I am waiting with bated breath for your response. No, not simply to the written word, but to the message of the love and healing power of God that I hope you have been able to hear and feel, way deep down in your soul.

I hope you have felt that message through all the things I have been blessed to learn about the power of God to heal and transform... things I learned after returning to Louisiana where I experienced the deepest healing I have ever felt in my entire fifty-plus years on this earth …

I have learned a tremendous amount in the decade-plus since returning to Louisiana, as I have experienced the deepest healing I have ever felt in my entire fifty-plus years on this earth …

For instance, I have learned through experience, as well as through revelation, that as a human being, you can be in pain that is intolerable and still find God. Indeed, He has met me in the midst of anguish, not always rescuing me from it but always making His presence known. What comfort this gave my soul!

I have also learned that not only will He comfort my spirit, but provide nourishment for my body. He has sent provisions – even as I cursed His name – through the help of others. On more than one occasion, He sent people like my friend, Elaina, to my door with bags of food. "I have heard from God, Jamie: 'If you love me, feed my sheep.'"

Sometimes He has worked through strangers, like the time at the grocery store when I didn't have enough cash to cover my groceries and a complete stranger pulled out a 100-dollar bill and paid for everything. I knew that this stranger's name was Jesus.

Most importantly, He has delivered me … miraculously and powerfully … from the throes of insanity. Remember the little dog chasing the butterfly? Or the flight attendant sucked out of the back of the plane? Those were just a couple of flashes of the insanity I experienced over the years.

How about when I accused Tom of poisoning me because I refused to swallow my medicine?

Or how about the time I shook my fist at God for a situation I myself, had created by leaving my husband to run off with another supposedly "God ordained" man?

But, ever faithful, forgiving, and loving, my God took me from the depths of all this insanity and made my mind right again.

He blessed me with knowledge of my illness and how my mind was being used against me.

He gave me the revelation during my hospital stay in Carson City General Hospital that not only was I there because I needed to be there, but also that those people in that hospital were a good representation of the very people He came to save — the brokenhearted, the downcast, the downtrodden; the afflicted. More importantly, I learned to accept that I, *too*, was brokenhearted, downcast, downtrodden; afflicted and that I, *too*, needed more of Jesus in my life.

Significantly, one of the most important parts of the healing Christ offered me so freely was the way he delivered me from hatred. I hated Levi, I hated Tom, I hated the entire Pastoral Staff of the church I attended in Carson City. I hated José, and I hated Shane and Teela. I, at times, have hated my father and mother. I blamed each of them at one time or another for my demise and/or the demise of my family. But as I have sought my Father's face I have come to learn and to re-learn that I serve a God of love and it is His desire that all may find forgiveness. This means that in His grace, I, too, need to extend forgiveness. That indeed was a challenge for me!

I had to plead with God to give me the strength to find forgiveness for all those who I had so deeply despised and wanted so badly to hurt. That forgiveness did not happen overnight. It took years of prayer and dedicating and re-dedicating myself to God over and over again. It took me being real with God and real with myself. But eventually I was able, for the most part, to forgive all of them.

And when the anger resurfaces from the memories of betrayal and abuse, I repent and choose to forgive… again. I am human after all and being human my heart is desperately wicked. It is only through the saving grace of Jesus that there is any of the good in me of which I speak. I struggle daily to be more like Jesus, squashing the ugliness of my flesh as it seeks to destroy my testimony.

I learned through that experience that the truest enemy we have is Satan himself. He is the father of lies. People are used as pawns in his game, and he is the author of confusion. He desires to steal, kill, and destroy.

Praise God I have a keen understanding of that now … though at times I still struggle with blaming the flesh and not the enemy. But when I fall victim to that trap, I quickly repent and give God praise for His gifts to me of discernment and enlightenment in my life.

Are you impressed with my God yet?—because there's still more!

Moreover, Christ has also lovingly and powerfully delivered me from the awful effects of disassociating. I was in such pain in my own tattered being that I attempted to put a distance between my inner soul and my flesh. I would disassociate from myself. That's why I created Lucrecia in my mind and experienced what would have been seen to the untrained eye as a dual personality. But it was, in simplest of terms, my maladaptive way of coping with the trauma I had experienced over and over again in my life. It was my way of putting some distance between myself and my tormented soul until I found healing.

In all goodness, Jesus has delivered me—from me. Oh yes! Yes, He did, and today, He still does. I have learned about Jamie, that she is very strong-willed and determined. That can work for me or work against me. And in so many instances, when my will has not been conformed to the *true* will of God (not what the enemy would have had me believe was the Lord's will), it has worked against me. The pain and the anguish that comes from the human heart when it has set itself like flint against the plans of God are sometimes easily overlooked at first. I know. I have been there, repeatedly, and if not for the grace of God, I will be there again.

Look back at the story of my life you have just read.

Go on, *look*!

How many times have I set out to make plans and failed to check in with God to learn if those plans were *actually* His will for me? Ohhhh, and how many times have I shaken my fist at God because *He* refused to yield to *my* plans, only to have God gently chuckle at me as He has allowed me to pitch my adult-sized tantrum, throwing myself onto the floor, pounding my fists, and thrashing my feet as I demand that *He* give in to *me?*

He sits there quietly, the loving, gentle Father that He is, and allows me to exhaust myself. Then He says to me, "Jamie come here and let's talk this over." As I reluctantly climb onto His lap, His arms lovingly and comfortingly embracing me, I can cry right into His shoulder and be reminded of His love and my frailty as a human. It is during these times that God has revealed to me,

"See — my plans for you are so much better than what you have planned for yourself.

"Trust me, Jamie. Trust that I am a good and My plans for you are good."

And in all sorrow, I repent for my tantrum and my strong-willed nature, and I wrestle with my flesh until it comes into submission to His will for me.

Still, I forget sometimes to submit my plans for God's approval, and still I shake my fist at God, and still I repent and ask God to forgive my desperately wicked human heart. And still, He does.

My Father has also delivered me from trust issues where the church is concerned. It hurt me and my children deeply when our church's staff in Carson City turned us away at the very time we needed them most. In fact, it took thirteen years before we all went to church together again as a family. But now I sing praises to my God each time we go because my *family — my husband and my children* — are there singing praises alongside me.

And God has healed and saved me through my beautiful children. As a mom, they believe I have saved them, but the truth is they have saved me from utter destruction more times than they will ever know.

God has delivered me from so much, but with everything He has delivered me from, He has replaced it all with something so much better …

In replacement of the many things, He delivered me from, God has given me the gift of love … for Him, for myself, and therefore, for others also. One of the first places I experienced that love was at Carson City General, where I understood for the first time, the depth of His compassion for those who suffer, which included me. I never knew a love so deep as when I found God in the psych ward of the hospital. He poured His love into my soul... for His people... for me. I felt such warmth as the love of Jesus flowed into my being. It felt like warm water being poured over me, washing me from the inside out, and removing the impurities which were meant to separate me from the love of God.

The love of my Father and His Son are like nothing this world has to offer. Even the purest of gold or the most radiant diamond pales in comparison to it. It is otherworldly and beautiful beyond comprehension to the human mind. It is something you have to feel and experience yourself to fully appreciate.

As I have stated and do again now.: I am so eternally grateful to my Lord for the love He has poured out over me and into me throughout the years. I am grateful that with each outpouring there was a re-awakening of my soul.

Yes, of all the gifts God has given me through this long, difficult journey to reach Him, love has been the greatest of them all. Nothing compares to this gift, nothing has more power to heal, nothing has more power to change. It is by the great gift of His infinite compassion that I have been healed and remain that way.

And it will be the only way you for you as well.

May you seek out this gift from God, and receive it.

Chapter 27

My Journey to Healing

While my journey to God began at the tender age of nine in Mrs. Joy's house in Ville Platte, Louisiana, it wasn't until sometime later that my relationship with the Lord would be instrumental in my journey towards healing. That healing process didn't really begin until twenty years later, as I endured being a patient in Carson City General Hospital.. Getting a formal bipolar diagnosis was the revelation through which I became painfully aware that I needed healing.

However, it wasn't until three years later, at age thirty-one that I began to aggressively search for healing. When Tom threatened to leave me if I threw my medicine away one more time, I realized that I needed to stop looking for some miraculous "instant" healing, where Jesus would just wave His hands over me and make all the anguish and suffering go away. No, the way I needed to be healed, the way Jesus wanted me to seek healing, was through those meds and the power of their underlying medical science that made them effective, the very science He had inspired mere mortals to use in order to create healing solutions

So why did it take me three years to finally get on the road to healing. If I am to be very honest, it was because I was in denial; I didn't want to face the fact that I was mentally ill. Instead, I wasted precious time. I sat around; I wallowed in self-pit. I ignored the words of Dr. Rizzle, who encouraged me to take my medications, eat well, exercise, and find a counselor. I ignored Tom's pleas to do the same. I ignored my inner voice telling me that things were not going to change unless I stopped being so proud and faced facts.

Day after day I ignored my mental health needs. At one point, I summoned the courage to do some research on bipolar disorder, chemical imbalance, and lack of serotonin. It didn't get me very far because I became overwhelmed and stalled out. For example, it took me one year to read an article on what the lack of serotonin and a chemical imbalance can do to a person. It was just a three-page article! I couldn't finish it because it was challenging my denial and I wasn't ready to face the truth!

But finally, I summoned inner courage and began my journey by facing reality. I read the article and I began to put my denial behind me ….

What did I learn from the three years I squandered?

Embrace knowledge … Embrace change … Embrace healing!!!

I learned my denial did nothing for me other than delaying the healing of my illness. It hurt me. It hurt my family. It took time from me and gave me nothing in return; nothing but more pain, heartache, and sorrow. I learned that I needed to face reality head on, with Jesus right by my side, and to believe that there was a way to healing —f I would seek it with my whole heart.

And that's when I chose to *take the first step!*

If you're in need of healing, *I implore you, take the first step!* Do it for yourself and your loved ones. Do it for the glory of God!

Once I braved taking that first step, it was easier to take the next, and the next, and the next...

Let me share with you the steps I took on my healing journey, which I am so hoping will help you heal.

Step 1: Admit that you need help.

If you're entertaining denial, please—for yourself and your family—find the courage to face reality.

Will it be hard? I will not lie to you. Yes! It will be hard. Will it be painful? Yes! It will hurt.

But the good news is, you're already in pain and on a path with no hope of the pain coming to an end. So why not take a step off that path?

Will it be worth it? Yes! Yes! Yes! It will be *more* than worth it.

The healing is worth the pain it may bring. But you can trust in the process. You can trust in God's ability to take you through the pain and to walk you through the process to find your healing.

The sooner, the better.

I am pleading with you! Don't allow the pain you are feeling now to control you any longer. There is help for you! Get out and get the **help**!

Is your world spiraling out of control? Are you feeling that you can hardly stand the thought of facing another day? There is help for you! Get out and get the **help**!

When you are using inappropriate coping skills, or self-medicating with alcohol or drugs, or even denying your condition with that teeth-gritting, *iron will* of yours to get you from one day to the next, don't suffer alone — there is help for you! Get out and get the **help**!

Is your family life suffering and are your friends becoming more distant than ever before? There is help for you! Get out and get the **help**!

When you can no longer stand the mask you are wearing and you are drowning in your own silent tears, trust in the process — there is help for you! Get out and get the **help**!

I had to accept my own frailty. I had to accept that it's okay to need help. I had to realize that no one was designed to be a lone island, not even me. No one was designed to walk through this journey of life without needing some form of assistance in the process.

I wanted to believe I was strong enough to pull myself out of the flooded pit in which I was drowning. I was too proud to ask for help. I wore a mask for years.

Can you relate to my words? If you can, may I suggest something?

Don't fight it. Don't give in to the temptation of merely surviving for another day. You may be thinking, "I am listening, Jamie. I can relate." Or "My mom is suffering; how can she find healing?"

I encourage you to embrace your journey or help your loved one embrace theirs and follow the steps I am giving to find the healing that is needed. There is help! Get you or them out and get **help**!

Before I go any further, let me encourage you to remember that the power of God is for you, your mom, your sister, your spouse, your child, your friend. God is on the side of all those who willingly reach out for His help, admit their need for help, and face it head on.

Step 2: Reach out.

I know from my own personal experience, reaching out can be scary. In fear, in panic, in horror, in pain, in desperation … I reached out. I admitted to needing help. I had to—because I needed the healing, and I didn't have the power to heal myself. It was bigger than me.

Yes, I knew the Lord. Yes, I had faith—but God chose to allow my healing to come over the course of many years and with the help of a psychiatrist, a pastoral staff, a counselor, the support of my friends and family members, psychotropic medications, and my personal hard work, sweat, and tears. My healing has been realized not only through faith and pouring myself out to God, but in trusting in the many ways and means He was placing in my path that would ultimately heal me.

My healing came from *working out the process before the Lord* and trusting Him to help me to take one step at a time until I was able to find remission.

Please understand that the truest healing will come from the throne room of God. I walk in healing and mental stability today. I believe with every fiber of my being that I have been healed by the hand of God. Yes, there is a process and yes, you have a part to play in it.

The apostle John reports in Chapter 9 of his book in the Bible, that even the man born blind, whose eyesight Jesus restored by means beyond today's medical capability—beyond human understanding—had a part to play in his own healing. The man was told by Jesus that he had to go to the Pool of Silom and wash the mud out of his eyes that Jesus had rubbed on them. "So, the man went and washed, and came home seeing." (John 9:7b)

Yes, I needed to go to my own Pool of Silom, which included my psychiatrist, church leadership, my counselor, and my friends and family and do what I was told to do: take the prescribed psychotropic medications, eat right, get moving and seek counseling.

But I need you to know that I never would have had the strength to walk through the process if it hadn't been for the Lord meeting me daily on my journey—as I walked. I also want to point out that my most profound healing came the day

I raised my arms in Mrs. Joy's kitchen and Jesus came to live in my heart as my Lord and Savior.

My spiritual healing is my most powerful healing. But aside from knowing that heaven is my home and my eternal destination, my flesh still has to submit to the process of healing, as prescribed by those who work so hard to help me. Yes, I had completely unraveled throughout the years. Some of that can be attributed to a toxic and unhappy childhood, some of it was my own doing, some of it was a result of being victim of others' actions, some of it was the emergence of mental illness during the turbulent teenage years of my high school experiences. Regardless of what caused the unraveling, I believe it was all within God's will and plan for my life. I know that … now. And whatever you may be experiencing in your life, you can *be certain that God has a plan for you*. You may already know that, but I just want to encourage you to hold onto that when your faith waivers, as mine has.

As I cried out to Him and in His wisdom, He seemed to tarry, I felt at times as if He had forgotten about me. But no! I have learned that He is so much bigger than that. His plan for me has included the pain, the suffering, the mental illness, the deception, the lies, the abuse, the mistakes I made, the trauma, the good times, the bad times, and everything in between.

God allowed it to happen so that I could come to know Him in a very profound way and so that I could come to know myself! I would never understand His power to save and cleanse had He not allowed me to experience this life and the particular trouble it brings. He did this for His glory and so that I could take my healing experience and offer it to you as a gift, a gift from God's throne room.

Step 3: Embrace the journey!

Rather than looking at the process of change with dread or fear, I urge you to look at it as an exciting opportunity; an adventure; a chance for better things to come both for you and your family.

One of the best books I have read is called *Who Moved My Cheese* by Spencer Johnson, M.D. It's a great read about finding the motivation to accept change. If you haven't read it, I highly recommend it. It's a short story but yields a very powerful message. I wish I had read it before I spent all those years squandering precious time and fighting the inevitable.

I hope that by reading the changes I needed to make, you have been inspired to change anything in your life that you aren't satisfied with.

If you are unhappy with anything in your life, don't wait another day *embrace change!*

Everyone's journey will look different. The first thing you need to do is to take inventory of what needs to change. Are you unhappy with your attitude? Are you unhappy with your mental stability? Are you unhappy with the way you eat, the way you sleep, the way you feel? Are you dissatisfied with your use of time, how you are handling work or parenting responsibilities?

I encourage you, be honest with yourself. It's essential to take a hard look at the things that need to be healed, whether they are internal (within yourself) or external (involving people and circumstances) and admit where you need help..

As you begin this process of embracing change, I encourage you to take an inventory of your mental health needs. There are many ways to do this, but I would like to suggest the following (use Internet search to access them):

- Beck's Depression Inventory (measures your level of depression, if any)
- PH Q 9 (measures for depression, if any)
- Burn's Anxiety Scale (measures your level of anxiety, if any)
- NICHQ Vanderbilt Scale [measures children for Attention Deficit Disorder (ADD), Attention Deficit Hyperactivity Disorder (ADHD), Oppositional Defiance Disorder, (ODD) or Conduct Disorder)
- Adult ADHD Self-Reporting Scale (measures ADD in adults)

Also, it is important that in conjunction with taking a mental health inventory, have yourself assessed by a trained clinician. Scales are designed to assist in the diagnosing of mental illness. They are a good place to start if you are wondering if you're suffering from depression or anxiety or a problem with attention deficit.

But remember that *step two* is reaching out. I suggest that you follow your inventory by contacting your local mental health agency and asking for the names and numbers of your local clinicians who take your insurance provider. You may also use the number on the back of your insurance provider card and ask for the providers in your area who take your insurance and provide mental health care.

Take your time and speak to the clinicians in your area and find one that you feel you would be comfortable with sharing your needs and pain. It will be somewhat uncomfortable, at first, but a good clinician will make you feel at home, as though you are sharing with your best friend over coffee.

Furthermore, the discomfort will dissipate as you engage in the process. Be encouraged, reaching out to professionals can be an important part of the process of change. This is something you may not have ever done before and as with most new experiences; change is a little awkward. Like the first time you went out dancing or water skiing, or snow skiing or even riding your first bike. It was a little awkward. But it becomes more natural with time and experience.

With your clinician, I suggest that you be forthcoming. Being a mental health professional myself now, I can vouch for the fact that the clinician can only help you by assessing the information you provide.

Keep in mind, your clinician is not a mind reader but:

- Will be listening for information that will be useful in helping you.
- Will not be searching for what is true and what is not true.
- Can only help as much as you allow.

Generally speaking, the initial assessment is the longest and probably the most awkward. Your clinician will ask a lot of questions: some personal, some medical, some to gather your history, and some demographic. These are all used in making an accurate diagnosis of your specific condition and then, finding the best way to assist you in healing. Let me assuage your concerns — no matter what the diagnosis, rest assured that there is help for you.

Making the diagnosis is simply a process of finding and organizing your symptoms into an understandable and treatable group with a descriptive word or phrase that collectively identifies the areas where you need help. It is the symptoms that are important. Your diagnosis' name, then, is simply a short-hand label for your specific condition, but it can also assist you in understanding where to aim your research. I encourage you to view diagnosing as a discovery and description tool to help you and your clinician define and pursue your healing process, much the same way a blueprint is used in directing a construction worker on how to build a structure.

After the assessment and as you learn about your diagnosis, listen to your clinician's recommendations. This is where I went wrong. I stalled out once I was diagnosed. It took me three, painful years to do research, educate myself on my needs, and work up the courage to proceed. Please, don't take this painful and wasteful route. Embrace your journey! Keep pushing forward! Put the recommendations into action right away, or as soon as possible.

If your clinician suggests:

- Reading material, do yourself a favor … read the material.
- A support group … go to the group and engage in the group.
- Weekly or bi-monthly counseling … attend the sessions and engage in the counseling process.

Yes, it will be awkward talking to a stranger about issues that are sensitive and private. But can I be real with you for just a minute? If your way of doing things (which is now probably comfortable to you) was working out for you, would you be hurting and in need of and seeking help? Probably not.

Albert Einstein once said: "Insanity is doing the same thing over and over again and expecting different results."

So … doing more of the same will only get you more of the same results. And if you want to get *different* results it's time to do things *differently*.

Notice, I didn't say *better*, I only said *different*.

A good counselor will help you to learn your symptoms, the triggers to your symptoms, and then help you identify coping skills that empower you to overcome your symptoms or teach you how to avoid them altogether.

For instance, maybe you have an anger problem. It will be vital to your healing to learn what causes you to be angry (your triggers) and how to cope with your anger or to avoid it (coping skills). Let me give you an example from my own life.

I used to stress over my financial situation. No matter what I did, each month my finances would have me in fits until one day I read a book on budgeting (a suggestion from my counselor) and it changed my life. I put a budget into place and learned to live within it. It didn't happen overnight, but it did happen.

I had to re-train myself and formed new habits. I learned to stretch my finances. I learned to eat off-brand foods rather than all name-brand foods, shop the sales, stick to a list at the grocery store, and put money aside for a rainy day. I learned to say no to snacks at the gas station. I learned to cook more and eat less frozen foods or take-out. I learned to set the temperature and leave it alone, using fans when we were hot and blankets when we were cold. I learned to enjoy activities that were far less expensive like movie night at home rather than going out to the theatre. I learned to pay my bills first and live off what was left rather than the other way around. I paid my tithes monthly and trusted in God to supply all my needs according to His riches in glory.

In short, I did a *different* thing which led me to a *better* result.

That is what the healing process is all about: making changes to your lifestyle. I have made some changes in every area of my life. I eat differently than I used to: I drink more water, eat fewer sweets, seldom drink alcohol, eat more fruits and vegetables and nuts, cook with olive oil, and purposely live a peaceful life.

I have learned to set boundaries and stick to them. I take naps every chance I get on the weekends. In my personal life, I distance myself from negative people and avoid people, places, or things that trigger my mental health symptoms. I avoid bars,

I avoid loud crowds. If I can, I avoid drama (drama-filled places, situations, or people), and I spend as much time as possible with the people I love. If I notice that something triggers anxiety or depression or even mania, I avoid it if and when possible. For example, I know that long road trips are a trigger for me, so I prepare myself mentally when we go to visit my husband's family in Texas (a three-and-a-half-hour drive). We stop along the way and eat ice cream and I take a restroom break or two. This breaks up the trip and allows me some downtime to cope with the anxiety of the long drive.

I listen to gospel music or Joyce Meyers on the radio or the country music station and that helps also. I refuse to allow my anxiety to dictate to me what I will or will not do. But I do work within my limitations, accepting that I am human.

I have also accepted that I need people in my life. I confide in my spouse when I am having a bad day. He is my rock here on this earth. He has been my anchor for the past decade-plus and I have learned to lean on him when I am weak.

I have also trained myself to listen to him when he tells me, "Jamie, you need to rest. You've had a hard day, now go take a nap." He knows me and he watches out for me. We do this for one another. He is a huge blessing to me, and God knew what I needed when he allowed us to meet. My husband is my biggest supporter on earth.

Yes, indeed, a good support system is essential to your process of making changes. You will need someone to speak into your life who can say, "Good job!" or "I am there if you need a shoulder to cry on." Or just someone to offer you observations of your behaviors and how you are doing from the outside looking in. We don't always have the most accurate picture of ourselves, and an honest support system is essential to find healing.

Check in with your support system regularly suggest that you choose three people in your life that you can trust enough to speak into your life, at any time, to give you advice or their observations. I have more than three. I listen to my sister, my children, and my spouse regularly, even to this day. I don't' always like what they have to say but I listen, and I pray about it, giving heed to their words of love and concern.

And don't forget God here. God, your Heavenly Father who has a wonderful plan for you and His Only Begotten Son, Jesus your Lord and Savior in whose name you can bring anything to the Father. Remember His Holy Spirit who dwells in you. What a support system! Consult these Three-Personalities-of-God-In-One through daily prayer and in their word to each of us, the Bible. Seek to be in the center of His will for you and seek to do—from there.

Attitude Towards the Process of Change

Please understand that change is not an event, it is a process, a journey ... to healing and wellness. Give it some time.

Remember, in general it takes twenty-one days to form a new habit and three to six months to break an old one.

Take a lesson from an old pro, post-graduate student—still in the school of hard knocks—it's easier if you learn to be a friend to yourself. When you fall and slip back into old habits out of frustration or force of habit:

- Repent of them before God and ask for His forgiveness,
- *Forgive yourself* for having fallen back into those old habits,
- Pick yourself back up again, dust your butt off,
- "Get to gettin," as my Grandma Hilda would have said, and
- Be quick to do all of these things.

It's okay to be human. It's the one thing we all have in common — our humanity, our frailty, our propensity towards making mistakes, and our need for a Savior. When you fall, once you've set yourself upright with God and yourself, and dusted your butt off again, review your actions.

Ask yourself, 'Where did I go wrong?' If you don't have the answer, ask your support system to help you to find the flaw in the plan and your actions, or talk to your counselor and ask them to shed some insight onto the subject. And be willing to make adjustments where needed.

Do this over and over and over and again, times twenty-five — or better still, "seventy times seven" as Jesus said. (Matthew 18:21-22 KJV) … Learn from your mistakes, without beating yourself up. Make adjustments; do it better next time. Keep moving forward and do yourself a favor, no matter how hard it is or how long it takes, ***don't quit the process!*** When you fall, fall forward. When you trip, trip forward. Whichever you do, keep moving forward. …

I have learned to trust in His will for my life when I fail and fall backwards. I am not perfect at trusting Him, I still find myself trying to reason (argue) with God and change His mind, as though I could or should. "God, can we talk? Can you please leave your throne and come and have a conversation with me? I am sure you will see it my way."

But I am much better now at recognizing my folly and I have learned to quiet my flesh and listen to the voice of God in my life. This has gone a long way to creating an appropriate "Attitude of Change."

I hope the three steps towards healing I have shared herein will be helpful to you. In addition to these, I have put together a workbook that goes along with *Lucrecia -Memoir of a Manic Woman,* to empower you, my reader, to take full advantage of these mental health secrets I have outlined here that I have learned over the years. I hope you will take advantage of this resource. It is, without a doubt, a passion of mine to ensure that you have everything necessary to walk in the healing I currently enjoy as a recovered mental health patient.

Walking in God's Peace

I am learning to surrender to His will. I am learning to walk in that peace that surpasses all human understanding by aligning my will with God's will in my life. I do this through prayer, communing with Him daily, and seeking His face regularly.

I pray that all my words have been helpful to you as I have laid my life open to you. Truly I suppose, my life has become "an open book!"

Please read it!

Please find yourself in it!

And, most of all, please learn from it!

Epilogue

So...what's up with Jamie today?

Thankfully, due to the Lord's amazing grace, I am still doing exceptionally well as far as my mental/emotional and physical health are concerned. In fact, I am counseling mental health clients forty hours a week, teaching them the principles I have outlined in this book. I am still in the process of undergoing supervision to become fully licensed as a Licensed Professional Counselor in the state of Louisiana.

I live with Brent in our home in Whiteville and we are the proud grandparents of six grandchildren, four girls and two boys. My children (except for my last son) all live within twenty-five miles of our home. Brent's daughter (my bonus daughter), Danielle, lives about forty-five miles from us. We all see one another regularly and enjoy spending family time laughing, loving, and making memories.

My oldest daughter, Tabatha (Tabby), has married the love of her teenage years, Ashton. Together they are making a wonderful life together and are the proud parents of two baby girls (Jordyn who is six and Josie who is three).

My oldest son, Jonah, works for a roofing supplier and distribution company. He has also met the love of his life, Tessa, and together they are happy as two people can be together. I love Tessa and am so blessed that she and Jonah found one another. Together they are serving God and planning for their future.

Gabrielle (my Doobie) is currently living with Brent and me. She is dating a young man (Walker) whom she loves. Together they are praying to see what the future holds for their relationship.

Benjamin (my Benji) still lives in Nevada with his dad. He is self-employed and sells furniture for a living at this time. I surely do miss him, but he was never a country boy and hated Louisiana. Therefore, I let him return home to Nevada when he was seventeen, to live with his dad in what he considers home. We talk regularly and it warms my heart to know that he is where his heart is happiest.

My first husband, Levi Guidry, the father of my three oldest children, has gone to be with the Lord. He lost his fight with cancer, three days after giving his life back to His Lord and Savior, Jesus Christ. He and I were not on speaking terms when he passed, but still I prayed that his suffering would come to an end, and he would find Jesus again for his sake and the sakes of our children.

My second husband, Tom Herbert, is living in Nevada with my youngest son, Benjamin. He and I do not speak, but I have no anger or ill will towards him.

Pastor Mickey Stryker and I are still fast friends and still communicate regularly. He lost his loving wife, Carmine, to cancer recently. How I do miss her. He is now remarried and has been blessed to find a wonderful God-fearing woman, Faith Stryker to join him as he serves the Lord Jesus.

My mom lives in the nursing home in Pine Prairie, about twenty miles from me. I see her weekly. She and I have a good relationship now and she is enjoying her time with friends she has recently made. It was a hard transition for her, but one that was necessary due to her ongoing struggle with diabetes.

My dad and I are still not on speaking terms, but I continue to pray that the situation will change someday through the healing power of Jesus.

I am still very much in love with my Lord and Savior, Jesus Christ! I spread His message of hope and healing every chance I get at home, at work, and in the community. My Heavenly Father has blessed me beyond my wildest dreams; I am eternally grateful for all He has done for me.

Life is good!

About the Author

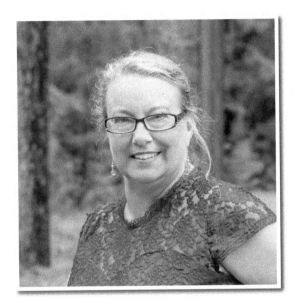

*J*amie B. Goudeau is a Christian author who was born and raised in a small community in south central Louisiana—the heart of Cajun country. Jamie is the blessed wife of her husband, best friend, and biggest fan, Brent Goudeau. She has four adult children and one bonus child and the proud grandmother of six grandchildren, who are a large part of her and her husband's world. Jamie enjoys fishing, camping, attending church with her family, counseling, school, and writing.

It is Jamie's passion to assist those struggling with mental health issues of any kind. She has overcome her own diagnosed bipolar I disorder with psychosis through hard work, favor, and strength from her God, along with the support from her loving family. Despite her mental illness, Jamie earned two master's 1 degrees from Walden University and is currently under supervision to become a licensed professional counselor in the state of Louisiana.

Jamie wrote this book to empower those who are struggling with "invisible illnesses" such as bipolar, to know that there is life after a mental illness diagnosis. It can be the platform to propel yourself — through hard work, perseverance, and Godly courage — to become all God has designed you to be.

Printed in the USA
CPSIA information can be obtained
at www.ICGtesting.com
LVHW061115161023
761155LV00036B/1224/J